David Gramling, Robert Gramling
Palliative Care Conversations

Language and Social Life

Editors
David Britain
Crispin Thurlow

Volume 12

David Gramling, Robert Gramling

Palliative Care Conversations

Clinical and
Applied Linguistic Perspectives

DE GRUYTER
MOUTON

ISBN 978-1-5015-1268-1
e-ISBN (PDF) 978-1-5015-0457-0
e-ISBN (EPUB) 978-1-5015-0447-1
ISSN 2192-2128

Library of Congress Control Number: 2018954425

Bibliographic information published by the Deutsche Nationalbibliothek
The Deutsche Nationalbibliothek lists this publication in the Deutsche Nationalbibliografie;
detailed bibliographic data are available on the Internet at http://dnb.dnb.de.

Typesetting: Integra Software Services Pvt. Ltd.
Printing and binding: CPI books GmbH, Leck

www.degruyter.com

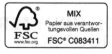

MIX
Papier aus verantwor-
tungsvollen Quellen
FSC® C083411

Contents

Part II: **Dynamics of the Interaction**

Acknowledgements

We thank the more than 250 patients and their family members who have agreed to share their experiences and perspectives with us for this study, as well as the more than 100 physicians, nurse practitioners, medical students, fellows, and residents whose work made this book possible. As co-authors, we are grateful for a brotherhood of patience, insight, critique, persistence, and willingness throughout the project – across the boundaries of discipline, method, language, and vocational identity. There are many colleagues in Palliative Care and Applied Linguistics around the world from whom we have learned in the process of preparing this book; we are grateful to you. Institutions that propelled this project onward at various points, through financial or intangible contributions, include the American Cancer Society that funded the study from which our data arose (RSG PCSM124655; PI: R. Gramling), the University of Arizona Office of Research, Discovery, and Innovation, the Ohio State University Center for Folklore Studies, and the Holly and Bob Miller Chair in Palliative Medicine at the University of Vermont. Suruthi Managarone and her team at Integra Software Services provided excellent copy-editing support. This book is dedicated to our cherished family and friends who continue to guide us and our work with their love, wisdom, and lightness.

https://doi.org/10.1515/9781501504570-201

1 Introduction

This book emerged out of the interactional work of hundreds of people talking with one another about living and dying in settings of serious illness. They are women and men, gay and straight, of color and white, Muslim, Christian, Jewish, Buddhist, Wicca, agnostic, and atheist, low-income and affluent, monolingual and multilingual, old and young. The questions and themes these speakers take up together range from the profound to the minute (see Bolden 2006, 2009, 2010) – and they do so under conditions of great duress, suffering, struggle, and distraction (Alexander et al. 2014). The interactional work these people do, for and with one another, is the work of emotion, understanding, spirituality, empathy, morality, comfort, expertise, logistics, nourishment, community, care, knowledge, humor, doubt, and imagination (see Stivers et al. 2011).

But this work is always also the work of conversation itself, where a range of participants – from physicians and nurse practitioners to medical students, family friends, and seriously-ill persons (Azoulay et al. 2000) – co-create an unpredictable fabric of conversational speech acts among them, which help or thwart the accomplishment of certain interactional goals and meanings in certain moments (see Clift 2001; Ford and Thompson 1996; Goodwin and Duranti 1992; see also Costello and Roberts 2001; Fisher 1995; Waitzkin 1991; Frankel 1984; Nowak 2011). Sometimes the expression of these conversational goals may appear vague and diffuse to an observing companion or researcher; sometimes these are stunningly precise, urgent, and incontrovertible. At times, participants' contributions to conversation refer to concrete clinical health realities; at other times, they have nothing to do with hospitals or illness whatsoever. Sometimes speakers' goals coincide with one another; more often they do not – or, at least, they diverge in consequential ways. On occasion, seriously-ill persons' desires and identities are misconstrued, or go unacknowledged entirely. Often enough, though, the collective talk 'in the room' succeeds in recognizing that "Deep inside you, there's a part of you, the most inner part, that's entirely free from disease" (Kushner 2013: 34).

1.1 Conceptual groundwork

We titled this book *Palliative Care Conversations* in the plural, so as to emphasize our belief that there is no singular, exemplary conversational model that ought to be emulated in settings of serious, life-limiting illness – contexts where multiple curative interventions have proven ineffective over time. There is no script, either for dying or for the time just preceding death. Of course, none of us – even those who specialize in communicating about alleviating suffering in end-of-life

https://doi.org/10.1515/9781501504570-001

contexts – has done *dying* before ourselves. There are many such potential models for end-of-life conversation, and much of that exemplary plentitude comes forth in this book, thanks to the work of the patients, families, and clinicians featured in the ten chapters ahead. Forming the living core of this book are over 50 clinical conversations (selected from a much larger, multi-site set of audio-recorded consultations), which involve more than 150 patients, family members, Palliative Care clinicians, and clinicians from other specialties like oncology and neurology.

Because this book is meant to encourage exploration as much as it may also advance particular claims, we present as much of the interactional sequence of each selected conversation as is possible within the constraints of a 250-page print book. Whereas other studies may excerpt conversational data more sparsely, so as to articulate evidentiary support for a given thesis, we two authors understand ourselves – within the occasion this book provides us – as facilitating open and multidirectional dialogue among a broader general research community, one that decisively includes our current readers. We want these conversations to be discussed, appreciated, and rethought, and we hope that such broader engagement with them will help strengthen and clarify the value of Palliative Care, a field of health communication that is just now achieving sustained public awareness in the United States. In the spirit of collaborating with our readers, we have found it useful to represent these conversations in as much of their complex sequentiality, prosody, and social embeddedness as was possible (Curl et al. 2006; Local and Walker 2008; Couper-Kuhlen 2001), while honoring the anonymity and integrity of the contributing patients and clinicians. (For readers new to the kind of conversational transcription style used throughout this book, we recommend any of the helpful summaries of "Jefferson's Transcript Notation" system, particularly Atkinson and Heritage 1984: ix–xvi). A short table of transcription symbols can be found at the close of this introduction.

Readers – whether nurses, physicians, linguists, or otherwise – may not have the time to read this book cover to cover. Of course, there are many resources available that model for clinicians best practices in health communication (Bernacki et al. 2014; Kurtz et al. 2004). There are also multiple handbooks on the market that survey applied linguistic and communication studies approaches to health and wellness (Hamilton and Chou 2016). This book was therefore conceived neither to reproduce those efforts, nor to replace them. What we have sought to do, instead, is to offer a random-access resource that allows clinicians and applied linguists the opportunity to drop into the arc of inquiry at various points, to benefit from what they can, and leave the rest – until they next have an opportunity to do so. We offer no systematic theory, nor a totalizing set of tools and outcomes.

Instead, we draw on the wisdom and experience of hundreds of patients and family members, and scores of clinicians, weaving a composite resource of settings and situations which may be of interest and of use to working professionals, engaged scholars, and invested policy-makers. With these readers in mind, we include at the end of each sub-chapter a list of cross-references that might help them trace throughout the book a particular thematic thread that appeals to them most at a particular juncture in their professional practice. For those who choose to read the entire book through, the introduction clarifies terms, principles, and methods of data collection and representation, as well as elucidating some of the broader societal and institutional contexts for Palliative Care. The individual thematic chapters, in turn, can function as stand-alone topical constellations that, we hope, offer discrete and useful case studies in actual health situations where dignity, relief from suffering, compassion, recognition, and mutual understanding are at stake.

We do wager that health professionals, when reading one or the other chapter, will resonate easily with the predicaments represented therein; we have chosen moments of conversation that are common but unpredictable, inherent but dynamic, profound but mundane. These moments of real-life communication between patients, clinicians, and families in settings of serious illness routinely outpace and outwit idealized models of what health care communication looks like. Oftentimes, patients and clinicians say things that seem at first quite inappropriate given the seriousness of the context, or they say things in forms of language that seem out of place. Some of the characteristic norms of polite conversation seem to be confounded – in part due to the physiologically compromised condition of the patient and the emotional distress of family members. Dynamics and conversational features that are often held to be highly normative, in a Gricean sense (1975), are stressed and dilated in Palliative Care settings. We hope that readers come away feeling that their own experiences, in such institutional health settings and in situations of profound distress (Alexander et al. 2014), are both vindicated and normalized by the cases presented here. In this sense, *Palliative Care Conversations* may serve to illustrate a continuum of practices upon which patients recognize themselves and their experiences reflected (Gramling et al. 2016a).

1.1.1 Foregrounding social interaction

In the chapters, we share more conversation and context in each instance than readers of medical communication research might expect, and doing so was an analytical choice as much as it was an ethical or explanatory one (Goffman 1964; see also Goodwin and Duranti 1992; Hymes 1972b; Schegloff 1997). The field of Conversation Analysis, emerging from the discipline of sociology in the 1970s, has shown us that it is often most wise to foreground what Emanuel Schegloff and Harvey Sacks in 1973 called "sequential implicativeness." Beach (1990: 608) glosses this universal dimension of human talk as "the ways in which a current turn-at-talk projects the relevance of a next, or range of appropriate and expected, next activities." In interaction, words mean not only their dictionary meanings, connotations, and associations; they also 'mean' sequentially, in specific relation to where they fall within the various events and projects "going on" (Goffman 1974: 46) within the conversation overall – before and after that particular word or phrase.

With such insights from applied Conversation Analysis (Antaki 2011b) and linguistic ethnography guiding the spirit of our inquiry, we have found – in the context of Palliative Care consultations, too – that a mere one or two turns-at-talk (Ford and Thompson 1996; Sacks et al. 1974) often cannot evoke for analysis and appreciation the multilayered web of tactics, anticipations, and preparatory efforts that participants are undertaking in a particular moment of conversation. Sequential implicativeness is an omnipresent phenomenon of naturally occurring human talk, and therefore also of Palliative Care talk – whether or not speakers' conversational goals are being expressed jointly or individually, overtly or deniably (Bilmes 1985; Frankel 1984; see also Goffman 1964; Hymes 1972b; Johnstone 2000; Sacks 1992; on 'medical conversation analysis' specifically, see Antaki 2011a; Antaki 2011b; Drew et al. 2001; Maynard and Heritage 2005; Heritage and Maynard 2006; Monzoni et al. 2010).

Instead of seeing conversational interaction as a serial syntax of enclosed mini-events, one after another, Conversation Analysts tend to focus intense scrutiny on answering the *relational* question "why that *now*?" (Bilmes 1985). In keeping this question-of-thumb central in the analysis, CA researchers are not so much inquiring about a participant's 'intentional' strategy, as we might imagine it based on what she says and does not say, but rather about how the talk in that moment both manifests and mobilizes some of the normative sequential resources of human conversation, as these have evolved over millennia (Bilmes 1985; Lee and Lin 2010).

For the purposes of this book, too, speaker "intention" is always a less relevant – because less ascertainable – domain for reflection than are the manifest resources of talk, to which participants and researchers alike have relatively unobscured access. As interdisciplinary researchers inspired by Conversation Analysis, we too believe that such an analytical commitment to sequential implicativeness, and the practical insights it adumbrates, can help make space for a particularly powerful kind of 'situated ethics' (Barton 2006; Barton 2007b; Mularski and Osborne 2001; Solomon 2005).

1.1.2 Paradigm challenges in medical communication research

In the main, however, health communication research in medical journals – some of which we have ourselves conducted (Gramling et al. 2013b, 2013c, 2015b,

2016a, 2016b) – does not opt for the resources of Conversational Analysis, pragmatics, stylistics, linguistic ethnography, and other kindred methodologies in Applied Linguistics, which train their lens upon the situated and sequential nature of conversational interaction. Indeed, the approaches that have predominated in our own previous work are those that identify human-coded conversational themes in order to test quantitative and interrater-reliable insights, by way of larger batches of aggregated conversational data. By way of these methodological pathways, human-coding-based studies reveal important, actionable results about the prevalence and distribution of lexically indicated features in end-of-life conversation – like sadness, optimism, hope, discord, or "prognosis talk" (sometimes shorthanded as "prog talk"). Human-coding methods are also able to bring forth for analysis aggregated evidence about non-lexical, interactional, and pragmatic features of talk, like silence, which are as crucial as are the words spoken (Bartels et al. 2016; Back et al. 2009; see also Carr 2006, Kulick 2005).

To be sure, such theme- and lexeme-based coding – as we have used it in the past and will continue to do so elsewhere – can be as patient-centered, nuanced, and ethically ambitious as any other approach to health communication can be. But, in this particular book, we've decided to forego human-coding approaches for the duration, and rather to "live with Manny's dangerous idea" (Levinson 2005): namely, that "social order is the *local* product of interaction" (ibid. 432, our emphasis), and not an elusive, external lever-system guiding interaction from without. Singular, micro-level, local, polysemous utterances from particular individuals – never to be repeated in quite the same way, nor in quite the same pragmatic orientation – are thus the critical resource to which we commit our attention in this study, believing as we do that each of those individuals is a complex, competent maker of order and meaning, no matter what form of suffering she may be experiencing at present. It is particularly meaningful, too, that these speakers are making meaning in a relatively new Palliative Care disciplinary-clinical setting that is itself being invented and reformulated, day by day, in thousands of other conversations such as these.

In Stephen Levinson's words, Emanuel "Manny" Schegloff's dangerous idea was that "instead of thinking of social institutions [like, for instance, Palliative Care] as organizing and creating the interaction that takes place within them, we should rather think of interaction patterns as engendering the very social institutions themselves" (ibid.). The concept 'social institution' comprises here not just brick-and-mortar buildings, hospitals, floors, units, and clinical disciplines, but also includes a range of socially, culturally, and politically enframed discourses like optimism, sadness, silence, illness, hope, and indeed also dying. As such, and particularly as regards our encounters with emergent realms of health communication like Palliative Care, we aim to heed

Stephen Levinson's warning that we ought not "drop lines into the interaction waters hoping to catch fish [we] have already labelled 'power' or 'gender', or the like" (ibid.).

Alas, research funding agencies tend to prefer that we do precisely this kind of pre-labeled fishing, even when such labels ultimately reflect a somewhat distanced vantage upon interaction and meaning in its social situation. Indeed, in our prior work, this kind of predetermined categorical abstraction often has been precisely the propositional foundation that allowed us to achieve the interrater reliability required by most large-scale granting agencies and national health care institutions. We thus conceived *Palliative Care Conversations* as a rare opportunity to focus our own analytic awareness upon complex interactional phenomena that might elude reliable coding – whether because these emerge by way of culturally or sociolectally variant speech genres and metaphorical repertoires (see conversations 5.3, 5.2, 2.1, 3.1, 5.4), or because the phenomena are based in interactional features that are neither thematic nor lexical on their face (see conversations 2.3, 9.3, 3.3, 6.3, 4.5, 6.1).

Throughout the book, we accordingly present half-page transcripts representing up to two minutes of interaction in each case, on the basis of which we offer pointed, local, and synthetic analyses about "what is going on" (Goffman 1974: 46), and about the social (and clinical) institutions that appear to be being made anew before our eyes (Levinson 2005: 432). In order to make good on this commitment, our transcription methods subscribe relatively closely to those that Conversation Analysts tend to use (Ball and Local 1996; Jefferson 1983), while remaining cognizant of what Bucholtz has theorized as the problematic "politics of transcription" (2000; see also Alexander et al. 2015; Ball and Local 1996; Jefferson 1983; Jefferson 2004).

We should note, however, that we are not Conversation Analysts in the true sense of that commitment. Our purposes in writing this book tend to have more to do with investigating the clinical setting of Palliative Care, and with the seriously-ill persons who take up its services, than with gathering evidence about the complex conventionality of human conversation itself. For this reason, our approach and methods tend to hew somewhat closer to 'theme-oriented discourse analysis" (Roberts and Sarangi 2005; Schiffrin et al. 2001) than to Conversation Analysis proper. Still, we hold the endeavor and traditions of Conversation Analysis in highest esteem, and our approaches here are significantly indebted to its decades-long commitments to examining interactional detail. Sharing longer transcripts has the additional benefit of making room for the exciting prospect that readers of *Palliative Care Conversations* will come to different, opposing, and additional insights about the data, beyond those we ourselves offer.

1.1.3 Listening to patients as complex subjects

It is a matter of greatest value to us as researchers to acknowledge that the thoughts, perceptions, and language these patients have agreed to share with us are among the last they were able to share with anyone before dying. With no less than grateful solemnity, we take responsibility for the fact that the audio recordings made for this research study are some of the last existing records of these men and women's living voices, of their thoughts on a range of questions, and of their embodied subjectivity in language. As will become clear, some participating patients become quite interested in the singularity and addressivity of 'their' recording, knowing as they do that it will likely reach readers of a book like this one (see, for instance, conversation 5.3). Along with everything else that is going on in the talk, patients sometimes use the occasion of the recording to speak implicitly to a broader listenership beyond their clinicians, their loved ones, and those immediately present in the room – a listenership that extends interactionally to the readers of this book.

Engaging as readers and researchers with these transcribed conversations is thus not only a critical commitment to improving medical communication in contexts of serious illness; it is also a direct and vividly moral act of listening to those who, in almost every case, have meanwhile died and become our ancestors. In the spirit of honoring the names by which these people are remembered by their loved ones, we decided not to give pseudonyms to patients throughout the book, but to leave them anonymous instead. The subsections of each chapter are also named using phrases spoken by participants in the interactions at hand, from which we then distill a theme or critical implications. When reading a subsection heading in the course of one of the following chapters, or in the Table of Contents, readers are interacting directly with an idea, judgment, or experience expressed by one or another seriously-ill person participating in this research study.

Lest the invitation to listen directly to these patients strike the reader as unduly abstract, we hasten to add that participants in this study are often overtly endeavoring to marshal our attention (as researchers, clinicians, and caregivers) in the hopes of changing the discursive, interactional, and institutional realities they have been experiencing. They tend in the most varied of ways to undermine long-held assumptions about asymmetricality and powerlessness in medical consultations (Pilnick and Dingwall 2011; Frankel 1990; Heath 1992; Gill 1998; Maynard 1991; Mishler 1984; Parsons 1951). Not only do patients and family members find tactical ways to level the relations of power in hospital settings – using inside jokes, initiation rituals, anarchic metaphors, and ingroup jargon seemingly designed to wrong-foot clinicians in their attempts to guide the course of the interaction (see, for instance, conversation 5.4) – patients also articulate a formidable repertoire of lay expertise (Sarangi 2001; on the discourse of expertise see Abbot 1988; Atkinson 1995; Beach 2001; Cameron 2008; Drew 1991; Parsons 1951).

1.1.4 Patients as language experts

Having spent a significant portion of their lives in and out of hospitals (see Ariss 2009), these patients' perceptions about health care interaction in general have often become sharp, assertive, differential, and granular. In equal measure, they notice, appreciate, undermine, and critique habitual manifestations of institutional behavior in ways that clinicians often find surprising (see Ajzen 1991). Because hospital-based end-of-life conversations usually reflect decades of previously experienced health care conversations, the Palliative Care consultation often becomes the most germane opportunity and genre for patients-as-lay-experts to share what they have learned over their ongoing journey accessing and appropriating health care. Consider for instance the stance taken by one patient featured in this study – a 56-year-old woman with a stage-four cancer who died just five days after this consultation. With a hypothetical example, she is trying to explain (to a clinician) why the ways clinicians formulate answers to her questions are so important:

> **Patient:** I listen very carefully to words. Because. [1.0] Ok, silly example. [...] Say: There's a concert on Sunday it lasts eight hours it's free it's it's a band that you hate. You think that this is a good... can we go? And the response would be: sounds like a plan to me. Is that a yes or a no? (3.0) Sounds like a plan doesn't mean yes we're going. It doesn't mean no we're not. It's just an answer.

By saying "sounds like a plan" is "just an answer," this woman in our study is pointing to how utterances are interactional, not just propositional. Affirmative, negative, hedging, and/or neutral answers *do* things effectively and in complex ways, beyond the ostensible information they convey. Even without knowing the exact interactional context prompting her elucidation above, readers will recognize how this patient is herself an ambitious connoisseur of interactional nuance. As a seriously-ill person in a hospital setting, she has had every motivation to observe and theorize the very nature of everyday language practice in her clinical environment – including its constitutive discourses of politeness (Brown and Levinson 1987), symbolic power, euphemism, pragmatism, paternalism, privilege, indirection, avoidance, conversational implicature (Grice 1975), condescension, speech genre, stylization, and other features close to the heart of Critical Discourse Analysis (Fairclough 1995; see also Antaki 1994; Curtis et al. 2002).

More often than not, we find that patients and families, while sorting out the implications of their own illnesses and prognoses, are simultaneously working to reconcile their complex and sometimes precarious cumulative experiences with the symbolic order of institutional health care language. They "listen very carefully to words," as the woman above puts it – perhaps because they have learned as persons with long-term serious illnesses that they *must* do so to get what they need. They accordingly develop a certain discursive agility within the symbolic order and organizational behavior of the institution (Ajzen 1991; Atkinson 1995), despite the frequently concurrent diminishment of their bodily and cognitive agility. While not all patients in the study express their theoretical insights as forthrightly as the patient above has done, most do often implicitly register their epistemic *stance* about various interactional features, even when they do not squarely claim the epistemic *status* of an expert about language, health care, or their illness (Pollner 1987; Raymond and Heritage 2006; Stivers, Mondada, and Steensig 2011).

Had the participants in this study *not* exhibited such detailed and attentive engagement with the situated workings of language in the clinical setting, this would have become a very different book. It would have been composed with different questions in mind and would have reached different results. But indeed, as the data will continue to show, Palliative Care conversations are a symbolic and practical occasion in which patients and family members do more than broach profound topics of life and death. They also seize upon the Palliative Care consultation as a prime opportunity to reckon with their experience of having been a seriously-ill person in a hospital setting and, when such a reckoning behooves them, to therapeutically divest from long-held stock slogans about the curative promise of health care – of overcoming adversity, of being a fighter, of soldiering on, of never giving up. Others double down on their investments in precisely these curative images and ideals. For us as researchers, this diversity means that we must apprehend Palliative Care conversations as an interactional setting in which multiple and often mutually adversarial layers of discursive framing are at work – layers that produce a unique imbrication among expressions of personhood, precarity, critique, politics, cosmology, recognition, freedom, unburdening, gratitude, uncertainty, institutional idiom, and truth-telling. The very interaction among these layers in conversation evokes, in turn, the complex historical positionality of the discipline of Palliative Medicine in the United States over the last several decades.

1.1.5 The concept of Palliative Care

The US clinical health discipline of Palliative Care arose in the 1990s as an institutional response to alleviate patients' and family members' suffering amid serious illness. Unlike biological phenomena of pain, suffering involves not only negative sensation and potential tissue damage, but a "perceived threat to the integrity of the self (both physical and psychosocial), negative affective quality, a sense of perceived helplessness, and perceived loss" (Chapman and Gavrin 1993: 7). While there are other medical specialties that excel at treating pain, Palliative Care is oriented among other things toward the complex problem of suffering amid serious, life-limiting illness. From the Latin *pallium* for "cloak," the adjective *palliative* has come to mean "alleviating without curing," as in placing a coat over a person shivering from the cold – a situation of suffering complicated by social, infrastructural, and physiological variables. Palliative Care clinical strategies can ameliorate features that cause both suffering and pain, while not endeavoring *primarily* to undo the underlying disease etiology. Scores of other medical disciplines are dedicated to curing disease, and they achieve this goal with varying levels of success.

In US hospital settings, the Palliative Care service tends to be the sole domain of clinical medicine where insights about dying, life-limiting prognosis, and end-of-life planning are at the heart of the clinical matter, and not just one eventuality in the course of curative disease management (Australian Commission on Safety and Quality in Health Care 2013; Australian Medical Association 2014; Bernacki et al. 2014; Chou 2004; Crippen 2008; Dy et al. 2015; Field and Cassel 1997; Hamel et al. 2017; Institute of Medicine 2014; Kavalieratos et al. 2016; Last Acts Coalition 2002; National Consensus Project for Quality Palliative Care 2013; Candrian 2013, Levy 2001; Yalom 2009). Several studies have shown other medical specialties to be somewhat, if not profoundly, averse to speaking about death and prognosis explicitly (Christakis 1997; Clemente 2005; Lamont and Christakis 1999; see also Sudnow 1967). Designed in part to address this death-averse discourse culture in hospitals, the new clinical discipline of Palliative Care board-certified its first class of specialist nurses in the United States in 2000 and of physicians in 2008. Since 2000, the US has seen at least a threefold increase in the number of hospital-based Palliative Care consultation teams nation-wide, amid continuous growth of formal post-graduate fellowships in Palliative medicine. Inevitably, this rapid growth has led to some adverse structural and labor consequences, including burn-out and understaffing within the growing discipline (Kamal et al. 2017; Kamal et al. 2016).

Palliative Care is however not a new concept. Alleviating suffering has always been a central concern for nurses and physicians in their everyday work with seriously-ill and suffering patients. Recognizing this historical continuity, Australia's National Institute for Health and Care Excellence uses the additional, inclusive label "supportive care" to characterize all clinical stances focusing on "helping the patient to maximize the benefits of treatment and to live as well as possible with the effects of the disease" (NICE 2004: 18). What has changed from the 1970s to today, alongside the underlying historical continuity among caregiver practices, is the pace of technological advancement and the availability of curative interventional techniques. Keeping people physiologically alive is simply much easier than it was in 1960 – and thus more complicated in its clinical, interactional, spiritual, and subjective ramifications.

1.1.6 The emergence of Palliative Care in the United States

While innovative success in isolating and treating ever more specific disease etiologies at the most minute level surged over the intervening decades, attention to actual prognosis, patient experience, and the complications immanent in the ever-expanding expectations about curability lagged ever farther behind. Treatment options abounded, and each newly available option reinforced a general promise to patients that they *can* be cured – a message that, by the sheer ubiquity and simplicity of it, exacerbated tendencies toward so-called "futile treatment" (Gallois et al. 2015: 657). Indeed, the Australian Commission on Safety and Quality in Health Care determined that a large proportion of people throughout the Western world die in acute care hospitals – whether or not they wish to – rather than at home or in hospice care (2013). Dying in protracted ways, and in the kinds of hyper-technological settings people had never imagined nor foreseen for themselves, was a newly endemic feature of post-modern life. One of the first in-depth histories of aggressive curability discourse emerged in 1999, with Nicholas Christakis' book *Death Foretold: Prophecy and Prognosis in Medical Care*, which addresses developments in the culture of prognosis over the historical period 1890–1970.

Outside the United States, clinicians, educators, and policy-makers had long been developing methods for caring for patients with life-limiting illnesses: including Cicely Saunders at St. Christopher's Hospice in South London, who was profoundly influential in founding the modern hospice and Palliative Care movement, the Canadian surgeon Balfour Mount, Tetsuo Kashiwagi in Japan, and of course the noted Swiss-American psychologist Elisabeth Kübler-Ross (for an international comparative survey, see Hamel et al. 2017). In the United States, hospice care had been introduced as a large-scale Medicare benefit in the 1960s, but by the 1980s it had become clear that many seriously-ill patients were going without the wide array of hospice-based options they were entitled to. Potential enrollees assumed that, because the Medicare entitlement required participants enrolling hospice to forego further pursuit of curative therapies targeting their life-limiting illness, "going with hospice" meant "giving up," and the uptake of hospice remained stunted and stigmatized throughout the 1980s and 1990s.

Where academic medical institutions were slow to fund research into these systemic socio-medical paradigm problems around curability vs. suffering, major initiatives like George Soros' Open Society Institute's *Project on Death in America* (1994) and the Robert Wood Johnson Foundation-funded *Study to Understand Prognosis and Preferences for Outcomes and Risks of Treatment* (1995) helped shed light on the need for new structures, models, and policies about end-of-life care. These large-scale projects eventually compelled the US medical establishment to acknowledge a need for Palliative Care as a semi-autonomous discipline, which achieved full board-certification status in 2008.

Most of the large-scale US medical research on Palliative Care since the 1990s has been concerned with cancer primarily (Epstein and Street 2007; Ferrell et al. 2017; Heft 2005; Sardell and Trierweiler 1993; Schenker and Arnold 2017; Slevin et al. 1996; Weeks et al. 2012; Lutfey and Maynard 1998), while diseases like dementia, AIDS, chronic obstructive pulmonary disease, heart failure, and multiple co-morbid illnesses remain understudied to date. Infrastructurally, Palliative Care research has focused most on academic medical center settings and *specialty* Palliative Care delivery (Ferrell et al. 2017), while much more research needs to be undertaken in community-based and *generalist* Palliative Care contexts (with specialist support when necessary). Seriously-ill people from rural or otherwise hard-to-reach areas will increasingly access specialty Palliative Care via teleconsult modalities in coming years, thus creating new structures and processes of conversation. These are some of the new frontiers in Palliative Care, now ten years into its official status in the US as a medical discipline.

1.1.7 The ascendency of Patient-Centered Communication

As the modern hospice and Palliative Care movements began to catch on in the latter quarter of the 20th century, so did new models of communication throughout health care institutions (Bigi 2011; Fisher 1995; ten Have 1991; Nowak 2011; Pendleton 1983; Roter 1977; Roter and Larson 2002). Up through the 1980s, physicians were customarily understood as experts who make decisions and then communicate them, with varying degrees of clarity, to patients. Rapidly emerging around 1990 were new conceptions of "shared decision-making" designed to honor patients' rights of self-determination and participation in medical treatment choices (Barton 2007b; Collins et al. 2005; Epstein and Gramling 2013; Fisher 1988; Gramling et al. 2015b; Bélanger et al. 2014; Norton and Talerico 2000; see also Robert Wood Johnson Foundation 1995; Slomka 1992).

Such early models of shared decision-making had the disadvantage, however, of basing themselves in the default image of an empowered, knowledgeable, energetic patient-as-rational-actor advocating for herself in negotiations with relatively pliant health care "providers". In good free-market style, patients were envisioned as consumers who survey the pros and cons of a given course of clinical action, usually choosing from a kind of à la carte menu of curative treatment regimens, and making informed decisions about which course to take. While such an ideology of choice-based health-care access may be persuasive and empowering in cases of discrete, curable afflictions, people suffering multiple, serious illnesses and their dynamically interacting symptoms are not particularly well-served by this model of consumerism. Palliative Care arose in part to deal squarely with these increasingly frequent and baffling physiological predicaments and with the specific communicative needs arising from them, which outstrip most consumerist models.

The 1990s rationalist-neoliberal recasting of the patient (and family) as health care "consumers" has continued its evolutionary arc toward increasingly flexible communication models (e.g. "Patient-Centered Communication"), which envision a range of roles that patients and clinicians responsibly play in meaningful conversations (Dwamena et al. 2012; Emanuel and Emanuel 1992; Epstein and Street 2007; Hesson et al. 2012; Institute of Medicine 2014; Jaen et al. 2010; Kinmonth et al. 1998; see also Korsch and Francis Negrete 1972; Korsch et al. 1968; Lee and Lin 2010; Slevin et al. 1996; SUPPORT Principal Investigators 1995). These roles are conceived as dynamic, and as driven by patients in their situated and changing context (Collins et al. 2007; Emanuel and Emanuel 1992; Gill 1998; Gill and Maynard 2006; Gill et al. 2010; Robinson 2003). Many patients referred for Palliative Care consultations come utterly exhausted by all of the responsible, participatory assessment-of-options they have been prompted to undertake in the face of increasingly complex and low-yield treatments, and this exhaustion only adds to the "wicked and intractable problem" of end-of-life decision-making (Raho 2012).

Seriously-ill patients have spent years and years being "on top" of their illness; they have become lay experts (Sarangi 2001) in their own right – in the language, contingencies, (un)predictabilities, and institutional affordances particular to their often-evolving disease(s). While rational contemplation of treatment benefits and risks may previously have felt empowering and encouraging for them, to many it often no longer feels that way by the time a Palliative Care referral is made. What often emerges, around the juncture of a PC referral, is not merely the need for a more complex menu of discrete treatment options, but rather a thirst for good holistic recommendations that comport well with patients' values (Bernacki et al. 2014). No matter what their opinion about patient-centered decision-making may have been in the past or in the abstract, Palliative

Care-referred patients often require something less free-market-driven. Suffering from extreme persistent pain, extreme exhaustion, aphasia, depression, shortness of breath, and medication-induced side effects that alter their sensory and cognitive realities, such persons' subjectivity and self-expression call for a different kind of communicative competence on the part of attending clinicians.

Just as this book does not promote one script for guiding good end-of-life conversations, neither does it underwrite any specific *a priori* conceptions of communicative virtue, or of ideal conversational roles and behaviors (Curtis and Patrick 2001; Curtis et al. 2001; Dwamena et al. 2012; Epstein and Back 2015; Field and Cassel 1997; Keeley and Jingling 2007; Kurtz et al. 2004; National Institute for Clinical Excellence (NICE) 2004; Nussbaum and Fisher 2009; Raho 2015; Silverman et al. 2004; Solomon 2005). We find value in allowing the patient data presented in these pages to guide our reasoning and reflection about "good communication," rather than the other way around.

One of the reasons we believe it is important to remain agnostic, or at least skeptical, about affirmatively adopting specific models of communication is that the discipline of Palliative Care finds itself up against various standardization pressures in recent years, amid which it is ever-tempting to export managerial idioms into the clinical sphere. (On such language and talk "from the top down" in other service industries, see for instance Cameron 2008.) These recent developments are explored in the following section.

1.1.8 Conversation as the "procedure" of Palliative Care

While there is an ever-present tension between the expert languages of health care professionals and the vernacular language of patients, there is also something of a rift between the procedural idioms of health care institutions, research funding agencies, and insurance lobbies on the one hand, and the vernacular clinical languages of everyday Palliative Care personnel on the other. Put another way, there is often as much of a divergence between clinicians' speech genres and the models that have been designed to regulate clinical work, as there is between the language of patients and the language of clinicians. One touchstone of this tension between clinicians' realities and health care management discourse is the relatively common slogan that "Conversation is the 'procedure' of Palliative Care."

We describe this innocent-sounding maxim as a slogan because the phrase tends to circulate readily in the world of health institutional management and research funding – but not necessarily so in the everyday practice of Palliative Care nurses and physicians. Still, it has succeeded in becoming a kind of guiding macro-level mantra about the discipline of Palliative Care. Obviously, there is something alluring on the face of this idea: that talking itself can be a primary, effective intervention in situations of serious illness and suffering, where even understanding what exactly "quality-of-life" might mean is profoundly difficult for everyone involved. The metaphor of conversation-as-procedure, of words that can heal, appears valuable on this substantive basis alone.

But the notion of interactional talk as the "procedure" of Palliative Care – equivalent perhaps to radiation or chemotherapy in oncological settings – is charismatic in health-care institutional discourse for a different reason than just those implied in a vision of 'healing words.' The phrase, additionally, *does* something – by angling to recharacterize Palliative Care in the terms of a recognizable institutional syntax. It outfits the young discipline of Palliative Care with an outward-facing stance, functionally equivalent to those taken by other specialties within the interdisciplinary hospital landscape (Kaufman 2005; Lupton 2003; Parsons 1951; Waitzkin 1991) and, more broadly, within health care political discourse and audit/accounting systems respectively. For institutional managers, this slogan means: everyone has a manageable, billable procedure, and Palliative Care's procedure happens to be conversation.

Despite the sloganistic and fiscalized inflections of this proposition "Conversation is the 'procedure' of Palliative Care," applied linguists and linguistic anthropologists may find the metaphor of the *procedure* appealing nonetheless, because it seems to attune to the performative sensibility of speech-act-based theories of language (Austin 1962; Austin 1970a; Austin 1970b). These social science and philosophical traditions hold that we always "do" things with our words, and that we do these more-or-less effective actions in institutionally specific fields of practice and under certain "felicity conditions" (Austin 1962) – never merely conveying disinterested information or describing realities with words unburdened of power relations. To communicate a life-limiting prognosis of "24 hours to two weeks," for instance, is never just to describe an evidentiary reality; it is always also to threaten a patient's face, standing, and personhood in some profound, or at least effective, way. Palliative Care clinicians know that there is no easy way around this.

One might then conclude, upon the admission of this core insight, that designing Palliative Care consultations with an awareness for the performative dimensionality suggested in the notion of conversational "procedures" will yield insights and practices that improve markedly on those available from the information-sharing or "constative" clinical frameworks of previous eras. In this regard, there seems to be some exciting and timely methodological resonance between medicine-based Palliative Care research and performativity theory in the social sciences, opening up opportunities for interdisciplinary insight on best practices.

1.1.9 Performativity and procedurization

But the current horizon does not exactly suggest such smooth interdisciplinary sailing in the short term. As general insight into the practical, implicative, and performative nature of language use seems to have been gaining traction in the ways health care discourse characterizes the Palliative Care consultation genre, this interest in performativity is itself being subjected to institutional instrumentalization—faster, perhaps, than it is inspiring research insight. The proposition "Conversation is the 'procedure' of Palliative Care" does not just acknowledge a sophisticated feature of language generally, it quickly serves to justify ways to monetize and standardize that consultation as a 'speech act' – transposing what Palliative Care clinicians have been doing for decades into the institutional category of the "procedure." Such a transposition has profound implications for hospital coding, noting, billing, and insurance reimbursement practices – and of course, meanwhile, for how seriously-ill persons experience clinical care.

Once some set of practices becomes a "procedure," such an interventional event is required to have relatively regularized components and respond to specific prompts from reporting tools. It becomes responsive to economization and rationalization from beyond the discipline, whether or not individual clinicians choose to heed these changing external directives overtly. Meanwhile, researchers and managers continue to seek understanding about what exactly Palliative Care clinicians are "doing" with their language, and what patients and families are doing in return. The tug-of-war between emerging clinical research insight into complex speech acts, on the one hand, and the managerial instrumentalization of language, on the other, is indeed one of the urgent and defining aspects of the present disciplinary moment in Palliative Care in the United States. For us, one of the primary indications that this book was worth writing has been the general zeal among various stakeholders to learn how, and whether, to replicate effective clinical conversations and their components.

Attempts to regularize the Palliative Care consultation have gained momentum since Jennifer Temel et al.'s 2010 article on "Early Palliative Care for Patients with Metastatic Non-Small-Cell Lung Cancer," which demonstrated for the first time that Palliative Care was not only a good thing for seriously-ill persons' quality-of-life (Antaki and Rapley 1996; Barton 2007c; Dy et al. 2015; Gramling et al. 2016a), but that it actually might *extend life*. Temel et al.'s 2010 publication was a watershed moment for administrators and physicians from other medical specialties, who for the first time apprehended Palliative Care as something plausibly beneficial and measurable for all their seriously-ill patients, not just those who wished to stop pursuing cure-oriented treatments. Grantors and national health policy leaders, for instance, became eager to establish exactly what the measurable "active ingredients" were for a successful Palliative Care conversation – not only so that they could enhance the effectiveness of those ingredients, but also so these could be standardized and disseminated (Dy et al. 2015; Epstein et al. 2015; Gramling et al. 2016a).

Several major studies on Palliative Care communication have been walking this tightrope between the primacy of local conversational practice (its unpredictable singularity, its striking procedural regularities, its diffuse rituals, and its thick cultural conventionality) and, on the other hand, the encroaching imperative to procedurize its "active ingredients." The Harvard-based Ariadne Labs, directed by the notable surgeon and author Atul Gwande, have developed, for instance, a checklist of components for "serious illness" conversations, while the Institutes of Medicine's 2014 *Dying in America* document provides similarly itemized "core components of quality end-of-life care." (On end-of-life discourse generally, see Barton et al. 2005; Chou 2004; Crippen 2008; Field and Cassel 1997; Iedema et al. 2004; Keeley and Jingling 2007.)

From a discourse-analytical point of view, Barton et al. (2005) have concurrently identified salient interactional phases of end-of-life discussions in intensive care settings, which they enumerate as: 1) openings, 2) establishment of traditional authority, 3) discussion of current status, 4) decision-making with holistic effect, and 5) logistics of dying. Barton et al. ultimately assert that, in these intensive care contexts, "Physicians [...] use a number of subtle discourse conventions to reinforce the lay understanding of terminal status of the patient and to reserve the determination of futility to the professional judgment of medicine" (Barton et al. 2005: 261); see also Aldridge and Barton 2007; Gallois et al. 2015). This critical observation leads Barton to suggest that intensivists tend to reproduce certain interactional and rhetorical conventions (i.e., "active ingredients") so as to achieve these goals. While the Institutes of Medicine's *Dying in America* views such active ingredients as a positive model to be practiced and sought, Barton et al.'s critical description seeks rather to reveal an unspoken normative purposiveness underlying the regularities of the consultation: asserting authority to compel consensus.

Thus, from both health-promotion/policy and from discourse-analytical quarters there have been attempts either to regularize (in the first case) or describe the conventional regularity (in the second case) of end-of-life decisional conversations (Gramling et al. 2016a). While the predictive patterns Barton et al. (2005) describe are helpful in describing how conversations tend to proceed in ICU settings, Palliative Care consultation since 2010 has diversified beyond the ICU setting and beyond the occasional *ad hoc* end-of-life conversation conducted by intensivists and oncologists. In this new disciplinary landscape, the implicit goal is no longer merely to establish consensus about the futility of further treatment (Schneiderman, Jecker and Jonsen 1996; Kaufman 2005: 29).

Indeed, in the United States, palliative medicine has only recently (i.e., since 2005) established a consistent presence in hospital settings, thereby distinguishing itself and its practices from end-of-life planning habits and conventions within Intensive Care Units (Ferrell et al. 2017; Lutfey and Maynard 1998; Angus et al. 2004; Barton 2015; Barton et al. 2005; Cassell 2005; Crippen 2008; Curtis and Patrick 2001; Curtis et al. 2001; Curtis and Rubenfeld 2001; Iedema et al. 2004; Kirchhoff et al. 2002; Mularski and Osborne 2001). It is thus important at the current moment to develop a specific understanding of Palliative Care consultations as they are led by Palliative Care specialists, who bring their own range of resources and questions, and to regard these as distinct from the occasional palliative or "EoL" conversations conducted by oncologists, general staff nurses, and intensivists in the course of their other duties.

No large-scale studies have as yet undertaken such a descriptive enterprise about Palliative Care specialty consultation interactions in the acute hospital setting. Proceeding with this in mind, we shall allow the features and the interactional details of these Palliative Care conversations to guide how, and whether, we might in future work distill a list of the components of the Palliative Care consultation. Many of these components we witness in the following chapters are emphatically patient-driven and emergent, and therefore do not submit easily to institutional guidelines or even descriptive typologies. The thematic chapters that follow are meant therefore to be speculative and hermeneutic, rather than inductive or programmatic as to the notion of the "active ingredients" of a Palliative Care-specialized consultation.

1.1.10 Palliative Care conversations as an evolving endeavor

In his 1973 essay on "thick description," the anthropologist Clifford Geertz reminded us that "certain ideas burst upon the intellectual landscape with a tremendous force. They resolve so many fundamental problems at once that they seem also to promise that they will resolve all fundamental problems, clarify all obscure issues" (3). The ideal of "good communication" has been one of these notions that appeals so generally and so charismatically that it seems to promise a solution to every mistake, every predicament, every form of difference – in health care interactions and beyond. We approach the data assembled here with an agnostic and exploratory stance toward "good communication."

It is not that we disbelieve the ideals that motivate professionals to pursue good, or better, communication, nor that we are in principle skeptical that such a thing exists. Rather, we believe that best practices in clinical conversations, particularly those involving serious or life-limiting illnesses, are sometimes counterintuitive, and must be earned through attention to real interaction rather than to abstract virtues. The pursuit of such best communicative practices, we believe, necessarily takes health professionals along a pathway that is anything but straight-forward, one that is populated not just with ideals, models, and beliefs, but with the critical, "thick" description of experience, and the nitty-gritty details of how diverse, actual people actually talk. In order to develop best practices of "good communication" based on conversational data (Bernacki et al. 2014), early-career clinicians may need to re-trace the work that others have navigated before them – for instance, in the conversations in this book.

Geertz confirms this:

> After we have become familiar with the new idea, however, after it has become part of our general stock of theoretical concepts, our expectations are brought more into balance with its actual uses, and its excessive popularity is ended. A few zealots persist in the old key-to-the-universe view of it; but less driven thinkers settle down after a while to the problems the idea has really generated. (1973: 3)

It is this period of settling down that, we believe, is currently upon us in the maturing health discipline of Palliative Care. We have sought, in *Palliative Care Conversations*, to earn our own understanding about "good communication" through an empirical acquaintance with the evidence and counterevidence: the ways in which patients with serious illnesses in hospital settings actually talk and have talked.

As funding for health communication research grows, so inevitably will grow the tendency to isolate codable features of conversations, so as to flag them in larger data sets and quantitative studies. Doing so may allow for important epidemiological research about the relationship between conversation features and patient outcomes. Yet we acknowledge the methodological problematic emerging from the fact that "communication epidemiology" currently tends to guide attention toward reliable, reproducible measurement of conversation features and, often, away from the kinds of interactional, prosodic, and implicative elements of conversation that are the bread-and-butter of applied linguistic approaches to meaning-making. If we do not take a granular and contextual approach to Palliative Care conversations now, future studies may overlook the centrality of discourse, indexicality, pragmatics, and sequential implicativeness (Schegloff and Sacks 1973; Levinson 2000; Antaki 2004; Beach 1990; Grice 1975; see also Frankel 1984), elements that do not submit to research methodologies that rely on thematic, lexical, or prosodic coding primarily. *Palliative Care Conversations* is designed as an initial wager in this endeavor, using evidence from patient experiences to establish larger qualitative-analytical repertoires and critical vocabularies that might inform future qualitative, and quantitative, work.

1.1.11 Learning from subtlety, counterevidence, and competitive framing

We understand that health professionals want to learn how to better engage in difficult clinical conversations about death and dying, and we share this desire as researchers and caregivers ourselves. Indeed, there is much to take away from the approximately 50 conversations we present. But we are unsure that searching out "best practices" is the most effective and useful way to approach these data. Rather than offering "how-to's," we hope these chapters provide thick descriptions that complicate immediate practical uptake and encourage deliberation on the specifics of the conversations from which they come. In being as attentive as we can to the minute, granular, and often profound features of human interactions amid serious illness, we often need to deepen into the peculiarities of the interaction in a way that will be at least provisionally inconvenient for building institutional procedure protocols and best-practices manuals.

Indeed, however, the patients enrolled in this study granted us the use of their language on the explicit premise that doing so would help future generations of clinicians and patients achieve better communication and clinical outcomes. The sustained and in-depth study of naturally occurring talk in its context of situation is, we believe, one proper way to receive the gift that they have given. By "in-depth" study, we do not mean 'multi-layered and comprehensive' alone. We also mean the kind of *critical* depth that risks threatening established values, questioning institutional orders, and revealing unstated norms and inequities. We seek to embrace and amplify counterevidence that undermines prevailing hunches and truisms about death and dying, health care, and good communication – if for no other reason than because such is the evidence that these patients have entrusted us with. We do hope that the insights in this book will have merited their trust and consent. We also hope that an arc of communication, and indeed of teaching and learning, will have been established from these hospitalized persons to future readers and researchers.

As we draw out the various moments in these conversations, we intend to do more than describing the surface-level relations and deciding whether they exemplify good or insufficiently good communication. We intend, even, to go beyond simply identifying the social actions that are taking place, often extraordinarily subtly, in these conversational encounters. Indeed, we hope to show why these matter – why they produce, alter, and effect outcomes for people. It is this hermeneutic axis between the granular and the consequential that guides our analysis, knowing along the way that these conversations are indeed each *end-of-life* conversations, both due to their explicit themes and their adjacency to the experience of death.

We believe, for instance, that speakers in Palliative Care consultations often introduce, concretize, and illustrate meaningful conversational projects (Levinson 1992) in oblique ways, and not just in overt, charismatic expressions. Often the granular, minute features of a conversation – those features that might elude usual notice or coding – can be among the most monumental. What is not said, what is said only with great difficulty, or what is half-said and then left unresponded to are often the keys to a persistent project in the conversation—one a clinician may be struggling to cognitively accommodate within her own spontaneous disciplinary, emotional, stylistic or analytical schematics. The conversations considered in this book are somewhat unique in the sense that, though the Palliative Care clinician is often hoping to engage in a type of conversation with the patient that brings clarity about the current goals of medical treatment, the patient may have a completely different agenda or "project" for the conversation. This means that these conversations abound with what the sociologist Erving Goffman (1974) called "competitive framing," in which it is possible for multiple participants to be holding a simultaneous conversation with one another, in which each of these participants may have a wholly distinct notion or conviction regarding what the conversation is "about."

In such a setting, the classic unidirectional public health model of *getting the word out* or *raising consciousness* about alternatives to aggressive curative therapies will frequently fall on deaf ears. Patients and/or their loved ones may be thoroughly invested in pursuing a different or opposing project: for instance, getting their primary care physician and their oncologist to communicate more effectively or, indeed, to figure out a way to ensure fewer unannounced visits from unfamiliar clinicians and personnel. Of course, fulfilling precisely these goals, and only these goals, could be *the best* outcome of a good Palliative Care consultation focused on ensuring quality-of-life and alleviating suffering – the suffering, in these cases, of logistical and communicative confusion, or the suffering of lacking privacy, companionability, and serenity. Misapprehending a patient's stance in the midst of a competitive framing (Goffman 1974) as evasiveness or denial, and seeking to remedy it through more persuasive messaging, misses the point that patients are often *competently* pursuing justifiable and important projects that are noncorrespondent with the projects of the Palliative Care clinician (Hymes 1972a).

1.1.12 The consultation as a dynamic genre

For these reasons, we approach these conversations not as exemplars of a series of core components, nor as ideal meetings of equals, but rather as a complex symbolic and social space in which multiple, conflicting, and incongruous projects are being pursued at once, under compromised circumstances. In such settings, power is not merely an expression of static institutional privilege and prestige, but an active plane of dynamics upon which participants may achieve and develop recognition for their interactional projects at any given moment in the conversation.

Indeed, successful Palliative Care conversations frequently rely on a clinician's competent ability to cede her own interactional project to the project of the patient, trusted other, loved one, or non-Palliative Care clinician. Getting to the physician's preferred "official focus of attention" (Goffman 1974, Beach 1995), e.g., the prognostic or goals-of-care decision sequence (Beach 1995), may need to take a back seat, momentarily or over an extended portion of the conversation. This is not merely a question of letting patients air grievances or get things off their chest. Rather, the clinician in these moments participates in engaging exactly what the patient's and family's project is, regardless of whether this project is expressed explicitly and coherently in terms the clinician readily prefers, or whether the project diverges or perhaps undermines the intended goals of a Palliative Care consultation altogether. We believe this de-centering of the self is a different clinical practice than to merely let a conversation go "off the rails" or "into the weeds," as we discuss in Chapter Five on "Irony and Rapport".

We describe the conversational genre considered in this book under the umbrella term of the "goals-of-care" or "decisional" conversation. A word about "genre" is in order. We draw on the Russian linguist Mikhail Bakhtin's conception of "speech genre," from his 1952 essay on the topic:

> Each separate utterance is individual, of course, but each sphere in which language is used develops its own *relatively stable types* of these utterances. These we may call *speech genres*. [...] We are given these speech genres in almost the same way that we are given our native language, which we master fluently long before we begin to study grammar. We know our native language [...] not from dictionaries and grammars but from concrete utterances that we hear and that we ourselves reproduce in live speech communication with people around us. We assimilate forms of language only in forms of utterances and in conjunction with these forms. (1986: 78–79)

For Bakhtin, neither languages nor genres of conversation are learned from rulebooks or in formal instruction. Official forms of linguistic prescriptivism come far too late in life to be as effective in shaping the way people speak as are their everyday, intersubjective social experiences of languages since birth, and perhaps even prenatally. In the study of genre, Bakhtin thus shifts the focus away from top-down models of instruction and adoption, and inquires into the ambiguous, off-record social spaces in which persons learn how to speak in certain ways as opposed to others.

A second claim Bakhtin makes above concerns the *"relatively stable type"* of utterances. Social spheres and symbolically organized spaces – classrooms, hospital rooms, medical units, discharge offices – develop their own stable forms for the spontaneous, unscripted use of language. This rather uncontroversial sounding claim has wide-ranging implications, as Bakhtin's idea of generic "stability" means that we do not get to opt in, or divest from, these forms of talk from one moment to the next. Participation in a given space – say, that of an oncological consultation – requires of patients, family members, and other professionals that they recognize and participate in the "relatively stable type" of conversation that tends to take place in that sphere. Certainly, this relative stability allows for play, give-and-take, and spontaneity. But these affordances of, for instance, the "oncological consultation" genre tend to be flexible precisely to the extent necessary for achieving the pragmatic goals and intentions inscribed in that genre. In this sense, it is the genre of the conversation – and not the conversing persons themselves – that provides and manages the logic of conversation. And yet, there is no genre without the conversing persons who practice it into social existence, as Schegloff pointed out. Giving up the illusion of full creative autonomy, recognizing the compulsory norms inherent in conversational genres, recognizing furthermore that these dialogic norms are the preconditions for conversational self-expression at all, and yet honoring the intractable variability and heterogeneity of human speech – these are among the basic axioms of Bakhtinian linguistics.

We describe the conversations studied in this book as "decisional conversations," as they are designed from the clinician's perspective to promote thought, dialogue, and preparation among family members and patients regarding "next steps" in their course of medical care (Azoulay et al. 2000; Bélanger et al. 2014; Kirchhoff et al. 2002; see also Korsch and Francis Negrete 1972; Korsch et al. 1968). Do they want to pursue curative/interventional measures at all costs? What does suffering mean to them? Are there current or expected tradeoffs in seeking longevity over comfort, which may be relevant to their definition of suffering (Chapman and Gavrin 1993; Epstein and Back 2015; Heath 1989)? Do patients want to be lucid and pain-free, so that they can enjoy their remaining days, weeks, or months with their family members? Do they want to eat a steak and drink vodka tonics, after weeks or months of hospital food? Do they want to see their cat? What do they want to smell? Whom do they want to see? What is bothering them the most at the moment? How do they rate their quality-of-life at present?

These lines of thought are "decisional" to the extent they are conceived around the collaborative, dialogical pursuit of insight and transformation on the part of patients and their loved ones. We do not call these conversations "decision-making conversations," because we do not presume that there will be decision made, nor that, in order for the talk to qualify for this genre, any action need to be taken. Rather, we assume that at least one participant in the conversation (whether the clinician, the family member, or the patient) is animated by the desire to promote some form of decision-making or transformation of thought and action.

1.2 Study data and methods

1.2.1 The Palliative Care Communication Research Initiative

The transcriptions presented and analyzed in this book emerged from the Palliative Care Communication Research Initiative (PCCRI), a study funded by the American Cancer Society and undertaken at two large medical centers in the United States (one in the Northeast and one on the West Coast) between 2013 and 2017 (Gramling et al. 2015a). Participants in these conversations include 240 hospitalized patients with advanced cancer, their loved ones and "trusted others," Palliative Care-certified physicians and nurse practitioners, medical fellows on one-year Palliative Care fellowships, primary "bedside" nurses, medical students and other learners rotating with the Palliative Care team on multi-week stints, fellows and physicians from other disciplines like anesthesiology and oncology, and occasionally nutrition teams and spiritual advisers. Out of 133 consented clinician participants, more than half were themselves students or learners in some fashion.

The Palliative Care Communication Research Initiative is an observational study (including no interventional experiments) comprising inpatient Palliative Care consultations as they naturally occur in the hospital setting. We restricted this study to the hospital setting because Palliative Care consultation in the outpatient context is comparatively newer, less frequent and highly variable in terms of reasons for referral. When a hospitalized patient was referred for a Palliative Care consultation, the accepting clinical provider used a PCCRI pocket eligibility card (as needed) to identify potentially eligible patients. PCCRI Study Staff assisted clinicians in determining eligibility questions or clarifications as they arose. Once the hospitalized person had met with a member of the clinical Palliative Care team, those eligible (or their immediate family members) were given a brief PCCRI Study brochure and asked whether they would be interested in hearing more about the study. (Patients who were actively dying – meaning that the clinical team expected that they would die within the next 24 hours – were not approached for participation.) If a patient lacked cognitive ability to consent for research and had a legally established

Healthcare Proxy, the proxy was eligible to participate (33 of the 240 participants were proxies). Patients or proxies who agreed to hear more about the study were fully informed by PCCRI Study Staff, consistent with informed consent procedures. Patients/proxies who agreed to participate signed a written informed consent.

With the patient or proxy's informed consent, PCCRI Study data (as represented in this book) were collected from eight sources:

1) the patient's hospital medical and administrative records;
2) a baseline questionnaire completed by the patient or proxy;
3) a baseline questionnaire completed by the Palliative Care clinician;
4) deidentified digital audio-recordings of the Palliative Care conversation;
5) a direct-observation checklist and field notes from the Palliative Care conversation;
6) an immediate post-consultation questionnaire completed by the Palliative Care clinician;
7) a post-consultation questionnaire completed by the patient or proxy;
8) an in-depth post-consultation interview among a subsample of patient/proxy participants.

Note that "post-consultation" in items 7–8 refers to the next calendar day following the first recorded conversation with the Palliative Care team, regardless of whether the Palliative Care team continued to provide care for the patient during the remaining hospitalization. All participating Palliative Care clinicians completed a baseline questionnaire about themselves once, at the time of consent. This questionnaire took fewer than 20 minutes to complete and collected information about the respective clinician's self-reported age, gender identification, ethnic and racial identification, religious affiliation, vocational training and education, clinical practice type, and clinical experience. Given our emerging interest in clinician mindfulness in fostering patient-centered communication, we included a shortened five-item version of the Mindfulness Attention Awareness Scale for the clinician to respond to. This clinician Mindfulness questionnaire included such items as "I find it difficult to stay focused on what is happening in the present moment," with six potential responses ranging from "Almost Always" to "Almost Never."

1.2.2 Participants and limitations

We observed and digitally recorded consultations with consenting participants at the two hospital sites of the Palliative Care Communication Research Initiative.

After obtaining written informed consent, the Study research assistant placed a hand-held recorder with a built-in multi-directional microphone in an unobtrusive location in the hospital room (usually on the bedside tray table). Prior to the Palliative Care clinician's entry into the patient's room, the Study research assistant initiated the recording and returned after the visit to stop the recording. (Participants were shown how to stop the recorder, should they wish to do so at any time during the visit.) Our approach provided high-fidelity recordings that allowed transcriptionists to hear even quiet voices amid clinical background noises, such as high-flow oxygen, intravenous fluid pumps, and heart-rate/respiratory monitors.

What we know from pre- and post-interview data about the participating patients in each conversation is their self-reported age, gender, racial and ethnic identifications (according to US Census Bureau categories). We also know their answers to the pre-interview questionnaire regarding their current state of mind, and their self-characterization regarding optimism/pessimism in the face of uncertainty (Han et al. 2011). We know the kinds of cancer and other diseases from which each person has been suffering, and how their illnesses have been treated in the past. Importantly, we also know how each of these patients in the Study fared medically in the six months after the consultation. In the majority of cases represented in this book, the person died within four weeks of the recorded interview.

Some of the limitations of our insights into these patients' experiences issue from the fact that the consent protocol allowed only for "up to three" visits, such that we were not able to follow their experience for a longer period of time – say, during a subsequent readmission to hospital. Nor did our consent protocol allow us to record end-of-life and goals-of-care conversations *conducted* by non-Palliative Care clinicians, for instance by oncologists or thoracic surgeons. When these other clinicians had occasion to join a group consult in the Palliative Care context, they do appear as participants in the recorded conversations. But we do not have recorded data from interactions, for instance, in which an oncologist and a patient *alone* are discussing a potential Palliative Care referral or comfort-care measures. As noted above, the study is limited to people with advanced cancer, who represent only 30–40% of the inpatient population at the sites where the study was conducted.

A further constraint on our results issues from the fact that some or much of the work introducing the concept of Palliative Care to patients and family members (what it is, what it means and doesn't mean, why the Palliative Care team has been called, etc.) may have occurred prior to enrollment, because the recruitment protocol required patients to meet a member of the Palliative Care team before being approached for participation. We designed the Study in this way purposefully, because attending physicians sometimes do not inform their patients when they decide to make a Palliative Care referral, and we did not want patients to learn first from a Study staff member (rather than from a trained clinician) that they had been referred for a Palliative Care consultation. Most often this pre-consent "first meeting" with a Palliative Care clinician was very brief, but we did not observe or record this interaction in the context of the Study. Though clinicians often then repeat and reformulate such introductory material when they arrive to consult (post-consent), the recruitment, consenting and enrollment process exerts an uncertain effect on the talk subsequently recorded for the Study.

Though the audio-quality of our data is good, we do not have access to most paralinguistic features of the talk, nor to multimodal, spatial, gestural, and visual cues. Nor were we able to enroll non-English-speaking patients and non-emancipated minors. Future studies will seek to expand the longitudinal reach of the data collection (i.e., following a patient for longer than three visits) as well as the latitudinal breadth of insight across the hospital landscape (e.g., including referral conversations with oncologists and impromptu Palliative Care volleys from critical care physicians in the midst of other clinical conversations, etc.)

In providing longer (i.e. half-page) transcripts of conversation, we do hope clinicians from various disciplines will take the opportunity to notice and identify aspects of their own practice to which they would like to devote more critical awareness. We encourage readers to jump around within the book, to use the various resources – including index, glossary, cross-references, and annotated table of contents – as a random-access resource of possible topics, questions, and bookmarkable concerns that may emerge from their own practice. At the end of the book, we have included a section "Thematic Questions for Further Inquiry," which helps readers to approach the conversations with specific themes, concerns, and questions in mind. In the following sections, we lay out the specific background and scope of this project, and how its research results will be laid out in the book.

1.2.3 Methods, protocols, and procedures

The umbrella project from which these data arise is a longitudinal cohort study designed to answer the question: "What are the features of Palliative Care conversations that lead to patient-centered outcomes?" What *we* envision as "patient-centeredness" is that the processes and treatments that constitute one's medical care foster those things that matter to the unique person who is seriously ill. In the setting of serious illness, treatments designed to slow (or cure) disease often have negative tradeoffs (e.g., nausea, fatigue, pain, spending more time in a hospital or other health care setting, financial costs, family time-off-from-work costs, etc.). What matters most to people in this context will differ vastly, as will how they evaluate their overall quality-of-life. Indeed, judgments about what matters most often evolve, the closer one is to dying (or perceives oneself to be). Accordingly, studying patient-centeredness in Palliative Care settings required us to collect meaningful data directly from patients about matters such as their perceived quality-of-life, their understanding about what to expect, how long they believe they might live, and whether they choose to express preferences about how "medicalized" they wish their health care to be in the last few weeks or months of their lives. (By medicalized, we mean how focused their care ought to be on disease management, as opposed to comfort and quality-of-life, if such tradeoffs exist.)

We designed our data collection methods to be of very low cognitive and interactional burden, so that even very ill persons could participate effectively when they desired to. We designed questionnaires in this way so as to avoid the kind of misleading findings that occur in clinical studies that favor "healthier" participants, who are able to volunteer time and energy to long batteries of questionnaires and procedural interactions. To the extent appropriate in each case, we sought to invite patients and their families to opt into the meaningful and dignified legacy of having participated in research that may improve health care communication. Hospitalized people whose diseases are not curable or substantially modifiable can sometimes feel isolated and stigmatized in a medical environment designed to eliminate disease, and they can quickly come to feel, under such conditions, that their opinions about health care communication are moot or extraneous. We did not wish to further exclude such potentially vulnerable and marginalized persons from participating in research, if they were inclined to help others.

The initial patient questionnaire immediately followed the informed consent procedures. To those who wished to participate, we posed only 20 questions (or, if the person lacked the ability to participate directly, we posed these same questions to her or his chosen surrogate). We limited the number of questions to 20 because our pilot testing of the research protocol demonstrated that an instrument of more than 20 items was perceived to be qualitatively more burdensome to patients and would discourage participation. Each question was formulated to address something not reliably available from other data sources. For instance, we did not ask patients directly about their age, type and stage of cancer, other illnesses, or their recent use of medical services, because those are readily available in the medical record. We did however ask patients about their racial, ethnic, gender and religious affiliations; global quality-of-life; bothersome physical, emotional, and spiritual symptoms; understanding of their illness, treatments and prognosis; and preferences for end-of-life care (Gill et al. 2010; Hagerty et al. 2005; Heath 1992; Heft 2005; Peräkylä 2006; Robert Wood Johnson Foundation 1995).

We structured each question based on the Dartmouth COOP (Cooperative Functional Assessment Charts) "field measures," which were designed specifically for ease of use in the clinical setting. Patient-participants were able to complete the questions in written form (via large-print paper questionnaire) or have the questions read aloud by the Study research nurse verbatim (on the interactional nature of questions, see Couper-Kuhlen 2012a; Heritage 2002; Heritage 2010; Huddleston 1994). During the pilot phase of protocol development, we tested and modified each question and the associated response options to ensure cognitive comprehension. The Study protocol provided for initial and ongoing training for the four Study research nurses, in order to maintain a uniform approach to question-asking and to limit any personal influences on patients' responses. Approximately two thirds of the study participants chose to have the questions read aloud. Neither completion rates nor distribution of responses differed for those who completed the questions on paper vs. those who requested they be read aloud. The duration of informed consent discussion varied based on the questions the patient or family posed about the study, but usually took fewer than 20 minutes. The 20-item patient questionnaire took an average of 10 minutes to complete.

Upon enrolling a participant, the research nurse left the patient's room but stayed in the general vicinity until the Palliative Care clinician arrived for the initial consult visit. The time between enrollment and first visit from the Palliative Care team ranged from minutes to hours. Upon the arrival of the Palliative Care clinicians, the research nurse informed the clinical team of the patient's choice to participate or not to participate and, in the former case, reminded them about the study protocol to which the clinician had previously consented. The research nurse then entered the patient's room ahead of the attending clinician to again request permission (i.e., to remind the patient about the Study and confirm his or her continuing interest in participating) and then, when appropriate, to place two digital recorders (one for back-up, in case of battery failure) with high quality multi-directional microphones in an unobtrusive location within 3–4 feet of the patient.

Although the research nurse was responsible for turning on and turning off the recorders (to emphasize that the attending clinician's role was that of a research *subject* rather than a researcher), all participants (patients, families, and clinicians) were shown how to turn off the recorder at any time if they ever wished to do so (though this never happened). If the room was not crowded, the research nurse remained in the background to passively observe any interactions that would not be captured on audio-recording (and then to enter these as a field note after the visit). If the room was crowded or no unobtrusive location was available, the research nurse stepped out of the room and waited outside until the visit finished to retrieve the recorders. For participating, patients and family members each received thank-you gift cards to a popular local grocery store or hospital café, valued at 10 US Dollars.

1.3 Using this book

1.3.1 Intended readers

The book is written with three rather distinct audiences in mind and is written in a style that is intended to include and recognize each of those audiences in as consistent and continuous a way as possible. This means that we are more careful than we would perhaps otherwise be to not overuse discipline-specific vocabulary, acronyms, or terms of art that may impede an unencumbered reading of the book. Of course, both the fields of health care and Applied Linguistics are flush with opaque, differentiated, and specialized vocabularies, and we hope to honor these languages without using them obtrusively ourselves. We recognize that a given word or phrase – say "comfort measures" in health care, or "translanguaging" in Applied Linguistics – is often a lightning rod for complex historical debates within the respective field about the underlying nature of a given category of human existence (here, "cure" and "language," respectively). We understand that the choice of one phrase over another can have immense practical, discursive, and institutional effects. With this in mind, we have tried to be as intentional as possible about terminology, affording it the power and role it holds in its proper context, while not assuming its universal applicability elsewhere.

The first intended readership for this book comprises clinicians, clinicians in training, and other health care professionals – whether nurses, nurse practitioners, physicians of various specializations, or Palliative Care personnel. We believe that the data presented here offer a unique composite sketch of the discursive and experiential universe of serious illness in hospital settings. While *Palliative Care Conversations* does not presume to make frequent clinical recommendations, we believe that important interventions and lines of thought emanate from the data themselves, when approached at the proper level of detailed awareness. By presenting (in most cases) more than a few turns-at-talk in a given conversation, we hope that clinicians will also be able to take away their own observations, identify similar scenarios in their past clinical work, and feel empathy and compassion with the patients and clinicians whose work is foregrounded here.

A second intended readership for the book is students and researchers of conversational discourse and language use, who may not have frequent opportunity to encounter such a spectrum of data in this setting of serious illness as they might like. Just as novel cross-cultural and intersectional situations of interaction reveal new aspects of conversation and language use, which may not have been evident in so-called monocultural or culturally homogenous settings, we contend that the context of serious illness calls attention to linguistic and conversational phenomena that, though universal in some respects, present in utterly provocative and singular ways in these conversations. To take one instance, Erving Goffman's concept of "face" (Goffman 1959; Morgan 2010; Defibaugh 2014) – and its subsequent uptake in the politeness theories of Penelope Brown and Stephen Levinson (1987) – gains new meaning when considered in circumstances of serious illness where one's very existence as a living person is imminently threatened, and not just one's symbolic value in social relations. While "face" is used most often as a metaphor for self or social persona, in Palliative Care settings a new level of poignancy and materiality accrues to "face." When a person is taking stock of the possibility that she may not live more than a few weeks beyond the current conversation, "face" is not just a social resource, it is also a primary embodied claim on physical and spiritual being the world, on existence, and on the collective recognition of one's being and having been.

For applied linguists, Palliative Care as a clinical specialty may be of particular interest because the 'decision-making conversation' itself is often considered the discipline's core 'procedure,' whereas other branches of medicine (from oncology to thoracic surgery) define themselves primarily through their (extralinguistic) curative interventions into the body. During their dialogues with patients, Palliative Care clinical teams therefore often embody and directly thematize an uncomfortably refracted or fractured image of the contemporary hospital's curative ambitions and imperatives. They both herald and highlight the ways in which repeated, incrementally invasive interventions, in pursuit of an elusive *status quo ante*, can lead to harmful effects to the patient – including excessive pain, misdirected hope, loss of autonomy, or the clinical inability to die a natural death (on discourses of hope, see Back et al. 2003; Benzein et al. 2001; Delvecchio Good et al. 1990; Dufault and Martocchio 1985; Eliot and Oliver 2007; Hagerty et al. 2005; Sardell and Trierweiler 1993; Thompson 2011).

A third readership for this book is those health policy-makers, legislators, institutional managers / administrators, and political leaders who, for one reason or another, have reason to be interested in the linguistic-interactional context of Palliative Care. Despite or perhaps because of its relative youth in the US institutional landscape, Palliative Care has quickly attracted attention from political leaders – ranging from electoral jockeying about so-called "death panels" in 2009 (Williamson 2012), to legislative acrimony around the Affordable Care Act of 2012 – and, prior to that, major jurisprudential deliberations from the 1990s onward about euthanasia and "right to die" initiatives.

To the extent that Palliative Care has been invoked in name or in spirit on these macro-political fields, its clinical purpose as a specialty has often been misconstrued or conflated with other, apparently neighboring arenas such as hospice care and/or physician-assisted suicide. Opportunistic as these conflations are in the political sphere, Palliative Care has nonetheless clearly become a proxy proving-ground for a range of freighted cultural, moral, and public-health dilemmas (Van Brussel and Carpentier 2012; Mouffe 2007). Indeed, indices of these debates regularly emerge in the course of clinical conversations with patients and families – in explicit, though ambiguous ways.

Of course, all of these readerships (clinicians, linguists, policy-makers) will themselves experience dying and the communicative activities around dying, and *Palliative Care Conversations* attempts throughout to recognize that "seriously-ill patient" is a category, experience, and status that the overwhelming majority of us will inhabit at some undetermined point in our lives.

1.3.2 Purpose, structure, format

We hope that this book will offer lay and clinical readers a series of practical scenarios, and an occasion to pause, contemplate, and identify. We believe the conversations shared here will lead many to recognize similar moments in their own practice – perhaps prototypical moments they have not noted previously, not seen described or investigated in detail, or familiar patterns that have felt important but whose importance was ambiguous, fleeting, or uncertain in the moment. Under current institutional conditions, Palliative Care conversations led by clinicians of other specialties are often not compensated sufficiently (financially or otherwise) for the professional time necessary to have them. Oncologists, critical care physicians, and others who choose to "have the talk" with families are often pressed for time and know that their efforts in doing so will not appear on any record of billable activity. Consequently, Palliative Care conversations in the daily flow of inpatient care often end up being uncompensated labor in clinical practice – valued implicitly and ethically, but nowhere registered in the disciplinary profiles of most health disciplines (beyond Palliative Care and hospice).

The main body of the book is divided into three parts, each consisting of three chapters representing a predominant conversational feature in each case.

Part I: Presentations and Introductions (Chapters 2 through 4) focuses on moments of introduction, presentation, and mutual recognition, in which clinicians and patients present themselves and their intentions to one another. In Chapter 2, we focus on the diverse ways clinicians present the medical discipline of Palliative Care to patients. Chapter 3 focuses on how patients bring their own lay (and, in a few cases, expert) knowledges about Palliative Care to bear on the conversation, and how patients and families query the nature, norms, and procedures of Palliative Care. This chapter highlights the way patients and family members follow up on, or investigate further, the details behind the clinicians' presentations of the discipline. Chapter 4, in turn, focuses on patients' own presentation of self, identity, history, and character in the course of the consultation.

　　Part II: Dynamics of The Interaction (Chapters 5 through 7) comprises three chapters focusing on rapport and irony in conversation, and the mutually reinforcing relation between them in the context of Palliative Care (Chapter 5); code-mixing and code-switching in conversations, including the dynamic mix of speech genres that participants use to negotiate with one another (Chapter 6); and how patients, for various reasons and purposes, ventriloquate and animate speakers who are not present in the current conversation (Chapter 7). **Part III: Some Components of the Consultation** (Chapters 8 through 10) focuses on three primary goals of Palliative Care conversations from the clinician's perspective: what we call "setting the table" for the consultation (Chapter 8); discussing and recognizing complex medical history, to whatever extent the patient considers this important to their current decision-making process (Chapter 9); and prognosis discussion (Chapter 10). Chapter 10 further serves as a retrospective summary on various features encountered throughout the preceding chapters.

　　Each chapter consists of a short conceptual introduction, followed by five to seven examples of conversations on the announced theme. We have chosen examples of conversations that demonstrate a diversity, indeed often a deeply divergent one, as regards the phenomenon the respective chapter seeks to adumbrate. For instance, Chapter 2 includes conversations presenting the discipline of Palliative Care in which the patient is a) already familiar with Palliative Care, b) deeply skeptical of Palliative Care, c) uninterested in discussing decision-making and quality-of-life topics whatsoever, d) frustrated with the hospital system as a whole, and e) eager to engage with Palliative Care decision-making. In almost all cases, each presentation of a conversation is preceded by a short profile of the hospitalized person, including age, self-identified ethnic, racial, religious, socio-economic, and educational background, self-rated quality-of-life over the past two days, self-rated prognosis vs. clinician-rated prognosis, etc. (on patient identity in conversation, see Egbert 2004; Eggley et al. 2017; Kagawa-Singer and Blackhall 2001; Fisher 1988; Fisher 1995; James and Clarke 1993; Oakley 1980; Todd 1989; West 1984a). In each case, we present one to four sections of each conversation (most often a half-page at a time) and make observations about each section of the conversation as it is presented.

1.3.3 The transcriptions

The conversations have been transcribed using Gail Jefferson's (1983, 2004) notation system, which indicates relative speed, volume, intonation, and pitch of the speech, as well as latching, overlaps, interruptions, pauses and pause-lengths, expressive inhalations and exhalations, and basic paralinguistic and non-linguistic features (see the table at the close of this Introduction). For the sake of readability, we have not represented the conversations phonetically, using instead US standard spelling unless a vernacular variation appears to us to have been particularly salient for the interaction. In Jefferson notation, it is important to note that punctuation (periods, commas, question marks, etc.) are used exclusively to indicate *prosodic* features of intonation, etc., and not for grammatical reasons. For those new to Jefferson transcription, we offer here a sample from one of the conversations.

MD: And ↑you <u>mu</u>st be Mister ____
1 Pt: I am ↑<u>he</u>! hh((laughter))
2 MD: ↑Nice to meetch you.
3 Pt: You ↓too
4 MD: ↑>Keep eating.=Is that <u>ice</u> cream?< hh
5 Pt: >Yes, this ice cream is [<u>good</u>]<
6 MD: [En↑joy] it=
7 Pt: =Right
8 MD: So,(.) ↑we're here with the <u>Pal</u>liative Medicine ↓Group=↓um, hh
9   (0.5) here to ↑talk (1.0)
10 Pt: Mm-hmm?
11 MD: Is that ↑<u>okay</u>?
12 Pt: Mm-hmm?

Note that in lines 10 through 12, the question marks denote not a grammatical question, but rather a rise in speaker intonation at the end of the respective word. To the best of our ability, we represent the interactional features of the conversation in a way that readers, who will not have listened to the audio recording of the conversations, can intuitively understand what is happening in a given moment of talk. For space reasons, we only include those sections of the conversation that are salient for observation, though we often include strings of talk that appear at first glance to be "off topic," (on topic-initiation, see Button 1988) and where some important interactional work is nonetheless taking place through minute conversational elements (Beach 1993; Bolden 2006; Bolden 2009; Bolden 2010; Clift 2001; Couper-Kuhlen 2004; Drummond and Hopper 1993; Gardner 2001; Heritage 1998; Jefferson 2002). In general, we refer to speakers as "physician," "nurse" or "nurse practitioner", "patient," "family member" (sometimes specifying familial relationship when possible), or "medical student". Doctors are sometimes distinguished as "attending physician", "fellow", or "resident", by which we indicate various levels in the training hierarchy, from highest to lowest institutional authority (see Collins et al. 2005). A table of abbreviations for denoting various speakers is included below in section 1.4.

1.3.4 Exploring conversational projects

As noted above, the three chapters in Part I focus on a) how clinicians present the medical specialty of Palliative Care in conversation, b) how and when patients and families query and question that specialty in conversation, and c) how patients and families present their complex selves to clinicians, while clinicians simultaneously co-create those selves, identities, and roles with them in the course of the conversation. Routinely, all three of these "projects" unfold in diverse and apparently disjointed ways within any given Palliative Care referral consultation with patients lasting more than ten minutes, and oftentimes more than one such project will be taking place simultaneously in a given moment of talk. In one moment, a family member may be seizing an opportunity to correct what he sees as an emerging (mis)characterization of his loved one, her history, and her perspectives, while the clinician, in the same moment, appears to presume that the topic at hand is explaining the role and purpose of Palliative Care as such.

Already in the 1970s, researchers of conversation were using evidence from face-to-face interaction showing how illusory it is for speakers (or retrospective analysts) to assume that participants in conversation ever truly share a common topic or theme in any given moment of talk (Goffman 1974). There is always some form of what Irving Goffman called "competitive framing" (Goffman 1974), even in settings where intimacy and rapport appear to be the primary tenor of interaction. This early insight from sociologists of language was not meant to paint a somber image of human communication, as always and ever "ships passing in the night," but to emphasize the complex and multilayered ways that human speakers tend to achieve understandings with and sometimes despite one another.

While participants in a conversation may sometimes share a similar version of a given topic – say, the idea that we are right now talking about "prognosis" and not about "symptoms" – these supposedly shared versions of conversational topic are typically inflected with divergent shades of investment and expectation, anticipated next sub-topics, specialized and vernacular vocabularies, and horizons of appropriate resolution.

We therefore generally take a cue from Conversation Analysis by speaking in the chapters of "projects" or "activities" rather than topics or themes of conversations, because designating a theme to a certain string of talk often obscures the discordance, centrifugality, and tension at work – phenomena that have been important objects of inquiry in recent Palliative Care research as well (Gramling et al. 2017; Butow et al. 2002). Subtly or ostentatiously as may befit them at any given moment, participants introduce (and often pre-introduce) new conversational projects, which they then seek to pursue and direct throughout the course of a conversation, whether or not that project appears at first glance to be contiguous or coherent, and whether or not they themselves would describe what they are doing in these terms. A project can, of course, go fully unacknowledged by the other parties to the conversation, without the conversation itself noticeably breaking down (Jefferson 2002).

The various projects in a given conversation – simultaneous, interwoven, or sequential as they may be in the talk – are often subtly corrective and performative. In introducing Palliative Care in a post-referral consultation with a family of a seriously-ill person, the Palliative Care clinician is, more often than not, demonstrably interested in correcting or pre-correcting misperceptions about Palliative Care, which she believes to be in circulation either in the present situation or in cultural discourses at large. Patients may equally be predisposed to seek to correct images, characterizations, details, and implicatures that they see emerging, or to clarify shared information – either in the current conversation or from the patterns they distill in their interactions with other, non-Palliative Care clinicians. All parties are thus interested in *doing* something particular, though not always intentional, with their self-introductions – of altering a salient narrative or of rerouting a narrative they do not believe is favorable to them. This regularity of conversation does not reveal human speakers to be cunning and strategic, as much as it shows that we are as a rule utterly competent at perceiving and adjusting to the implicative contributions of others, in the moment of their emergence (Levinson 2005; Sarangi and Roberts 1999; Schegloff 1991; Boden and Zimmerman 1991; in medical talk, see Frankel 1984; Gill 1998).

For this reason, introductions are not straightforward in the genre of Palliative Care consultations, nor ought they be. There are aspects of Palliative Care as a medical specialty that profoundly unsettle the normative historical prerogatives of the hospital as an institution, which is to cure disease. In intimating that medicine can and should do more than just curing disease – i.e., that it should alleviate suffering and ensure comfort and quality-of-life in serious illness – is a surprisingly controversial position to take, and this fact, though most often unthematized as such, is palpably reflected at all levels of talk within the data we present and analyze in these chapters. Throughout, it will therefore be just as important to grasp what various speakers are trying to *do* in a given moment of talk, as it is to understand *what is meant*. Chapter 2, "Representing Palliative Care" focuses therefore not only how clinicians present the medical specialty of Palliative Care to patients and families, but investigates what it is that they are seeking to achieve interactionally in those various presentations.

Though we will necessarily also consider how patients respond to these presentations, Chapter 3, "Querying Palliative Care" takes as its primary purpose an investigation into the ways in which patients speak back to, and question, the presentations that clinicians have offered them. Lest the word "presentation" suggest formality, we emphasize that these conversational projects of introduction and presentation take place within the normal, ordinary flow of conversation, not at any heightened or formalized distance from everyday interaction. Nonetheless, readers will notice particularly in Chapter 2 a preponderance of clinician-led conversation, in which physicians and nurse practitioners (Defibaugh 2014; Fisher 1995) speak more, hold the floor for longer, and benefit from patients' and families' forbearance and noninterruption in ways that suggests that a particular ritual of exchange is indeed being observed.

1.3.5 Our co-authorship

We decided to write this book together collaboratively, knowing that our different training, experience, and conceptual vocabulary would persist even amidst our dialogues while preparing this project. One of us (Bob) is a medical physician board-certified in hospice and Palliative Care who also holds a doctorate in public health and epidemiology. One of us (David) specializes in literary/cultural studies and applied linguistics. Both of us straddle, and treasure, our own trajectories of multi- or interdisciplinary training and investment; we each individually participate in at least two disciplines that find themselves often in productive conflict with one another: public health and hospital medicine on the one hand, cultural studies and applied linguistics on the other. Coming together to write *Palliative Care Conversations*, we each first needed to countenance our own internal interdisciplinary positionings, in order to prepare for the methodological dialogues we would undertake with one another.

Large-scale, interdisciplinary projects like this book are somewhat rare, perhaps because trust between medicine and the social sciences – let alone between medicine and the humanities – is difficult to establish and maintain (on efforts in the 'critical medical humanities', see Whitehead and Woods 2016). While medical humanities initiatives continue to bloom at research universities and elsewhere, these endeavors are sometimes undertaken at a distance from actual clinical work, and particularly from clinical work with seriously-ill patients and their families. Working clinicians have good reason to be choosy and guarded when deciding which non-clinical researchers to invite into their professional spaces, and federal laws are designed to be abundantly cautious in ensuring that patients' dignity, anonymity, and privacy are not impugned in the research process.

When interpretive social scientists are invited to be observers in clinical settings, they often do not have access to the complex institutional vernaculars that shape clinical care, communication pathways, and hospital hierarchy (Chabner 1996; Mishler 1984). This sometimes leads non-clinical researchers to apprehend certain discrete linguistic practices or habits at face-value, when they may be best understood from within the complex performative context of hospital communication logistics and discursive order. Sometimes things are said because they legally must be; other times they are said because a certain institutional protocol requires that questions be answered in a certain way or in a certain order for charting, billing, or compliance reasons. In this project, we treat these facts and features not as unfortunate constraints on the meaning-making process, nor do we attempt to bracket them out of the human interactional frame. We rather treat such normative constraints on conversations as both a constitutive feature of the talk and as one of the topics of contestation within the talk. Patients and clinicians all have opinions – whether latent or manifest – regarding hospital procedure. Oftentimes the implicatures that enliven and complicate the conversations we present in these forthcoming chapters are directly tied to the participants' comfort or discomfort with the institutional and material scripts they have been assumed to be subscribing to at a given moment.

Meeting for a common purpose, we discovered that the relationship between our respective disciplinary-conceptual maps was not hampered by absence and deficit at the level of vocabulary, as we first suspected. Medicine uses the word "rapport," just as often as linguistics does. Health professionals have as many ideas about "good communication" as do experts in intercultural pedagogy. Rather than discovering the absence of a certain key concept prized in our own customary research vocabulary, when searching for it in the practical sphere of the other, we found ourselves most often in the "What-*you*-(all)-mean-by" stance. David needed to learn when it was appropriate to speak of a "stage" versus a "grade" of lung cancer; Bob needed to wade into the dicey affair of differentiating "linguistics" from "applied linguistics" and delimiting both of these from "communication research" in the United States and elsewhere. Translating conceptual vocabulary across disciplinary frontiers can become an end in itself – and a heroically analytical one at that – but we had other purposes in mind. This meant finding ways to set aside purely translational work and accept the co-presence of often non-correspondent analytical foundations in our co-authorship. This is, after all, the experience for hospitalized patients too, who bring their own vernacular tools to an institutional setting populated by multiple, and often internally conflicting, expert discourses.

As co-investigators, we needed to come to terms, together, with the fact that medical and health sciences have their own intellectual lineages around "communication" that do not necessarily overlap with those prevalent, indeed presumed, in applied linguistics. Likewise, humanities and interpretive social sciences disciplines have certain diverging presuppositions about "culture" and "language" – let alone about ethnicity, race, health, gender, power, institutions, death, and the individual – which may cloud our ability to apprehend cognate concepts that are historically at home in medical and health disciplines. In the push toward interdisciplinarity over the 1980s and onwards, each macro-discipline (medicine and applied linguistics) seems to have succeeded in setting up, domesticating, and institutionalizing a certain heterotopic version of its respective other. Medicine and nursing have their own 'domestic' discourse about "communication sciences," while applied linguistics has built its own set of frameworks for health care discourse. This chiastic discovery may prompt researchers to summarily "bridge the gap" through remedial terminological reconciliation, but this gesture often overestimates individual speakers' ability to translate among the practical spheres that motivate the reconciliatory desire. Indeed, we sought to honor the durable intersectionality of the human settings we set out to study, precisely by allowing, for instance, words like "rapport" to carry all the social heteroglossia proper to them, rather than requiring a single, authoritative meaning.

1.4 Table of abbreviations and symbols

Throughout the transcripts, we use the following abbreviations to describe the speaking participants:

Dt: (Patient's) Daughter
Fel: Palliative Care medical fellow (traditionally holding an MD or DO degree)
FM: (Patient's) Family Member
Fr: (Patient's) Friend

MD: Palliative Care attending physician
NP: Palliative Care nurse practitioner
Onc: Oncologist
Res: Palliative Care medical resident (traditionally holding an MD or DO degree)
Son: (Patient's) Son
SiL: (Patient's) Son-in-law
Sp: (Patient's) Spouse
Uk: Unidentified Speaker

The following symbols are loosely based on Gail Jefferson's (2004) transcription system:

[text] Bracketed text shows overlaps with another person's speech, which is also bracketed

=   an equals sign at the beginning or end of a word means that a next speaker is "latching" onto that word, i.e., not allowing for a pause to take place between their contribution and the prior contribution. Speakers can latch to their own contribution at a "turn relevance place" or TRP, thereby holding the floor and preventing interruption.

CAPS   capitalized text is shouted or otherwise very loud speech

-         a hyphen at the end of a word or syllable indicates an abrupt break-off of the vowel or consonant; often a glottal stop

°°   text within is spoken quietly or whispered

><   text within is spoken faster

<>   text within is spoken slower

hhh   expressive exhalation

.hhh   expressive inhalation

:::   colons elongate the sound immediately prior to them

___   underlined text is emphatic, but not necessarily louder or higher in pitch

(0.2)   pause of 0.2 seconds. Note: pauses are measured to the nearest 0.2 seconds elapsed

(.)   a micropause of less than 0.2 seconds

( )   surrounds unclear or difficult-to-hear words

↑   indicates higher pitch in the following syllable or syllables of talk

↓   indicates lower pitch in the following syllable or syllables of talk

,   indicates a moderate rise in intonation, but does not mean the end of a grammatical clause

.   indicates strongly descending intonation, but does not mean the end of a grammatical sentence

?   indicates strongly ascending intonation, but does not mean the end of a grammatical question

Part I: **Presentations and Introductions**

2 Presenting Palliative Care

In this first thematic chapter, we analyze six naturally occurring, face-to-face situations in which clinicians present or re-present Palliative Care as one among multiple specialties and clinical roles in the overall hospital-based treatment of serious illness. "Introducing" Palliative Care is ultimately not an adequate descriptor for this conversational genre, because "introducing" presumes that patients and families are not already somewhat or quite familiar with the word, aura, or implications of "Palliative Care." Often, during a conversation days or weeks prior, patients' oncologists have shared their own understandings of Palliative Care and outlined what it can offer that oncology perhaps cannot. It is often on the basis of these non-PC-initiated descriptions of Palliative Care that patients gain a first explicit profile of the specialty, though frequently they have heard of it from previous hospital visits, family experiences, the Study consenting process, or other ambient cultural discourses. The conversations presented in this and other chapters clearly indicate that patients and family members rarely fail to take some meaningful epistemic stance on Palliative Care early on, based on what they know from other sources (on epistemic stance, see Beach and Metzger 1997; Delancey 2001; Drew 1991; Eagan and Weatherson 2011; see also Goodwin 1987; Jones 2001; Goodwin 1987; Lindström and Weatherall 2015; Chafe and Nichols 1986). Sometimes, as we will see below in conversation 2.3 for instance, the epistemic stance patients and families take about Palliative Care serves multiple interactional functions, including bids for status recognition.

Accordingly, it is perhaps more accurate to speak of the central theme of this chapter as "presenting and re-presenting Palliative Care", rather than "introducing" it. Such a project of re-presentation is necessarily more complicated than enumerating a frontal definition *tabula rasa*, as re-presenting entails for the clinician all of the following interactional mini-projects: *distinguishing* Palliative Care from ostensibly similar care philosophies like hospice, *justifying* the appropriateness of a Palliative Care-based discussion *at this time, describing* how and why this particular ensuing conversation has been initiated or requested, and *articulating* how Palliative Medicine as a specialty sees and understands itself generally and in this instance. Each of these four components of the "re-presenting" project has its own range of dynamic sub-components, and each of these brings with it, or "implicates," an intricate discursive micro- and macro-history that the patient and clinician loosely share. (By micro-history, we mean the cumulative experiences of the individual as they relate to health and illness; by macro-history, we mean the broader social discourses that have shaped and attended the course of their experience with illness thus far.)

https://doi.org/10.1515/9781501504570-002

Articulating how Palliative Care as a health specialty sees and understands itself is thus no straight-forward affair of showing patients a hospital badge and moving on to the business at hand. Nor is it merely a matter of conveying top-down talking-points about the clinical functions that Palliative medicine offers to seriously-ill persons, i.e.:

- an *extra layer of support*
- *symptom management*
- pharmacological, ergonomic, spiritual, and social strategies to *reduce suffering*
- *improving quality-of-life*
- helping families continue to make (often very difficult) *goals-of-care decisions*

Each of these five primary offerings by which US-based Palliative Care customarily self-identifies in its outward-facing materials (brochures, policy platforms, institutional profiles) is itself the result of decades of refinement, counter-distinction, reflection, and redirection in the face of public misconstrual or umbrage. One notices, for instance, that the words *death* and *dying* are not generally mentioned in the specialty's written materials, and even the phrase "end-of-life" is used only in a constrained and specific way (Lutfey and Maynard 1998). This regularity is indeed reflected in the naturally occurring conversations we share and analyze below.

As this book is focused on living conversations, we will not fixate overlong on the historical processes by which Palliative Care came to the custom of introducing itself in the ways it does in US hospital settings. Historical overviews are widely available (Australian Commission on Safety and Quality in Health Care 2013; Australian Medical Association 2014; Bernacki et al. 2014; Chou 2004; Crippen 2008; Dy et al. 2015; Field and Cassel 1997; Hamel et al. 2017; Institute of Medicine 2014; Kavalieratos et al. 2016; Last Acts Coalition 2002; National Consensus Project for Quality Palliative Care 2013; Curtis and Rubenfeld 2001). Rather, what we hope to demonstrate in this chapter is the contextual complexity that surrounds the project of "re-presenting Palliative Care," and how that complexity reveals itself in unique and naturally occurring interactions in hospital settings. We have observed a number of complicating themes that affect and structure the way the project of introducing Palliative Care tends to unfold in the settings we investigate:

1. **Provenance:** It is often unclear to patients and families who exactly initiated the Palliative Care referral, and why and when they did so.
2. **Patient Ambivalence:** Even if patients and families are aware that another physician has made a Palliative Care referral on their behalf, they are sometimes ambivalent about the timing, necessity, and/or purpose of that referral, and it often becomes necessary for the Palliative Care clinician to re-justify the

referral. Initial expressions of ambivalence are not so much directed toward Palliative Care as a specialty, but towards its seemingly random insertion into the overall sequence of clinical rounding among other specialist visits. (In the main, Palliative Care-referred patients are being regularly visited by representatives of more than three clinical specialties already.) As such, a patient or family member might be eagerly awaiting an expected or promised visit from a particular oncologist or primary care physician and is therefore less than enthusiastic to speak with the Palliative Care team about a topic they do not view as highest priority (on interdisciplinary and intergroup language in hospital settings, see Gallois et al. 2015; Hewett et al. 2015; Watson et al. 2012).

3. **Discipline fatigue:** Patients are not necessarily interested, at first, in being introduced to a new medical discipline – complicated as their health already is by an often-unmanageable range of clinical participants, by complex physio- and pharmacological symptoms affecting their recall and information retrieval, and by sheer exhaustion at managing hospitalized life from the standpoint of a seriously-ill patient. In the course of introductory conversations like these, Palliative Care's ultimate goal of alleviating logistical and physiological burdens is not easy for patients to square with the concrete *interactional* fact of being imposed upon by a new stranger representing a not-quite-familiar specialty with a quizzical name.

4. **Clinician ambiguity:** Palliative Care referrals from oncologists, for instance, are often tinged with an ambiguous mix of motivations – ranging from the referring clinician's desire to expedite and bolster health care delivery (a "the more, the merrier" approach), to clinicians' worries about staffing, scheduling, and shift-change dynamics on weekends, to truly sincere investment in Palliative Care as a specialty. For instance, one oncologist might make a Palliative Care referral because the weekend is nearing, and she wants another layer of clinical supervision for a seriously-ill patient while she is off, though she is fully invested in the likely curability of the patient's cancer. Meanwhile another oncologist will refer a similarly ill patient to Palliative Care because she believes she and her clinical team have truly exhausted effective curative measures and are potentially entering into the realm of "futile treatment" (Gallois et al. 2015). The nature of such divergent motivations in each case is often not expressed either to the Palliative Care team nor to the patient herself.

5. **Symbolic positionality:** Palliative Care often conveys ideas that are unfamiliar, if not adverse, to the predominant curative discourses of the hospital setting. Casting doubt on the curative promise of the hospital is already dicey symbolic terrain, not merely when *patients* are expressly committed to the ongoing maintenance of this curative promise, but rather because hospital discourse is always already premised upon it. It is of course possible to

imagine a hospital whose idiom is not exclusively that of the cure, and which pursues a broader ideal of care as that kind of support that can "nudge another toward wholeness" (Moore 2018: 57) without necessarily eliminating their disease, but this is not currently the state of US hospital discourse. Misgivings about curative discourses – whether on the part of clinicians, patients, or family members – are often already marked as potentially inappropriate conduct and therefore against the implicit rules of hospital discourse as a symbolic field – i.e., as "giving up" the game (Antaki 2011a, Atkinson 1995; Barton 2004; Barton 2015; Barton et al. 2005; Herndl and Nahrwold 2000; Sarangi and Roberts 1999). Building from the legacy of Talcott Parsons in the sociology of medicine, Pilnick and Dingwall (2011) refer to such behaviors of being "inappropriately sick" as a potentially scandalous violation, not just of the hospital's symbolic order, but also of the socio-institutional order of society at large (see also Chabner 1996; Mishler 1984; Kaufman 2005; Lupton 2003; Parsons 1951; Waitzkin 1991). Palliative Care, a heterotopic mirror (Foucault 1984) of the hospital's most deeply held presumptions, finds itself at the center of this precarious symbolic territory.

While the first four of these factors complicating the project of "re-presenting Palliative Care" might be remedied in future by better referral mechanisms and more streamlined coordination of multidisciplinary care, the last, socio-anthropological component cannot be remedied without profound paradigm changes in the self-understanding of the hospital as an institution. Because of the PC specialty's symbolic marginality in this broader self-understanding of the hospital, "introducing Palliative Care" is always in some way performative rather than merely descriptive, in that it has a transformative effect on the implied position of the patient within the hospital. These features can, we believe, be traced throughout actual conversations. It is this analysis to which we now turn.

2.1 I'm going to be a silent partner here

In this first conversation, which appears transcribed below in several sequential chunks with our analyses interwoven, a Palliative Care physician is attempting to present the idea of Palliative Care to a patient and his family. We propose the following general questions for readers to consider with us, in this and subsequent conversations:

1. With what kinds of language does the clinician seek to join the pre-existing community among the patient and family members, and what are the demonstrable effects of the way in which the clinician seeks to do so?

2. How do clinicians structure the clinician-initiated presentation of Palliative Care, using certain forms of personal deixis (*I* vs. *we*, etc.) as well as images of group membership ("team", "from the", "with the", etc.) (see Anderson and Keenan 1985)?

3. Is the presentation of Palliative Care tailored to the clinical situation of the patient, or does the clinician presents a broader picture of the specialty and then perhaps move on to elucidate its applicability to the particular patient's situation?

4. How do these conversational designs – practiced, spontaneous, or unintended as they may appear to be – elicit certain responses from patients and families, and why do they appear to do so?

This chapter focuses more than the others that follow on a clinician-initiated genre or project, namely on "re-presenting Palliative Care," which often occurs toward the beginning of a post-referral consultation conversation with a patient and/or family. Hence, by some necessity, the strings of talk we present here in Chapter Two tend to be heavy on clinician talk, in the sense of air-time distribution among physicians, patients, and family members. As with all of the conversations extracted in this book, we first present a brief profile of the hospitalized person in a standard form outlined in the book's introduction.

The patient in this conversation self-identifies as an 80-year-old white man and as financially secure, reporting graduate-level education and no religious affiliation. He has been diagnosed with a stage-four cancer that has not yet been biopsied. He believes he is "very unlikely" to live for a year, while his clinician-rated survival prognosis is two weeks to three months. In fact, he continued to live for 34 days after this interview, which means that both his and the clinicians' prognosis estimates were ultimately accurate and correspondent (on prognostic concordance and discordance, see Gramling et al. 2017; see also Horne et al. 2005; Jones and Beach 2005). This person considers his end-of-life goals as "comfort over longevity," and he rates his "global" quality-of-life over the previous two days – physical, emotional, social, spiritual, and financial – as a zero out of ten. The following portion of talk occurred during the first visit of the Palliative Care team, at the beginning of the recorded conversation. The clinician speaking is a Palliative Care physician.

1 MD: And ↑you <u>must</u> be Mister _____
2 Pt: I am ↑<u>he</u>! hh((laughter))
3 MD: ↑Nice to meetch you.
4 Pt: You ↓too
5 MD: ↑>Keep eating.=is that <u>ice</u> cream?< hh
6 Pt: >Yes, this ice cream is [<u>good</u>]<
7 MD: [En↑joy] it=

8 Pt: =[Right
9 MD: So,(.) ↑we're here with the <u>Pall</u>iative Medicine ↓Group=↓um, hh (0.5)
10   here to ↑talk (1.0)
11 Pt: Mm-hmm?
12 MD: Is that ↑<u>okay</u>?
13 Pt: Mm-hmm?

Even in this short extract, the physician-initiated talk displays a number of features worth our sustained attention: a) social joining, b) blended personal deixis, c) mixed vernacularity, and d) overt metadiscursive markers. *Social joining* is achieved as the physician not only requests that the patient "keep eating" the ice cream in line 5, but also inquires about the ice cream, which prompts the patient to make the encounter's first independent propositional (substantive) and axiomatic (value-conferring) declaration, "This ice cream is good." With this declarative assertion, the patient is following up on his light-heartedly overformal self-staging "I am *he*!" in line 2, where he intuitively selects an elevated tone befitting Shakespearian drama or diplomatic negotiations (on 'doing formality', see Atkinson 1982). Through social joining, rather than floor-taking, the clinician recognizes that the patient desires to be regarded as the principal autonomous agent negotiating the interactional space on his own behalf. Indeed, this status design will be borne out by the patient's subsequent selection (below) of a commercial or business negotiation sociolect ("silent partner" in line 16 on page 52, and "relatively short timeframe [...] available to me" in line 25 on page 52. It is worth noting that his frank and businesslike expression about expecting a "relatively short timeframe" was borne out as accurate, as he lived 34 days past this conversation.

The clinician's recognition of the ceremonious, diplomatic status the patient has designed for himself in line 2 above prompts the clinician to recalibrate the relative value of the incipient themes of the conversation. For instance, the clinician acknowledges that the goodness of ice cream may indeed be just as important in the scheme of things as is the physician-initiated goal of "presenting Palliative Care". Though the physician clearly has no intention of tabling his own project entirely, he will nonetheless extend more than nominal deference to the existing order of priorities in the speech community he is now joining. In this way, the physician indicates his willingness to join a social space where another topic might be taking precedence, and he seeks thereby to accommodate himself to that order – a gesture that appears to be well-received, as the patient immediately returns the token "ice cream," offered by the physician, augmenting it with a deictic shift from "that" to "this."

The physician uses further deictic resources to nuance the project of re-presenting Palliative Care in line 9: namely, that *"we're* here *with* the Palliative Medicine Group." This is what might be called an affiliative, proximal self-introduction, rather than a frontal, distal, or identarian introduction. The physician leverages situational legitimacy from the blended facts of his belonging to an established social entity (see Couper-Kuhlen 2012b; Drew and Walker 2009), while accounting for that entity as kind of omnipresent collective rather than a delegating body. That is, by choosing "we're here *with* the" rather than "we're here *from* the," the physician avoids the symbolic intimation of having been dispatched as a representative *from* some external force, a characterization that can evoke popular cosmological images of "the grim reaper," or political images of "the death panel" (Williamson 2012).

In concert with these tactics of social joining, the physician apologizes preemptively (below), threatening his own positive face by drawing attention to his lack of immediate face-familiarity in line 2 with the various family members in the room.

```
1   MD:   ↑All righty (.) I think _____'s gonna get some chairs for us, ↓°so°
2         And- I'm ↓sorry, how do you guys °know°-
3   Dt:   ↑I'm his daughter
4   MD:   >You're his daughter< =°Okay°
5   Dt:   And that's my husband.
6   MD:   And that's your hus-=↑All right=↓Just like to know, >you know<, who's
7         who.
8   Sp:   I'm the wife.
9   MD:   hh >And you're the wife.<
10  Dt:   ↑Really? hh ((laughter))
11  MD:   ↑I figured ↓that,
12  Sp:   ↑I'm the spouse. hh ((laughter))
13  MD:   Okay (.) All righty= Well >by the time we< get the ↑chairs (.) let me tell you
14        a little bit about what I ↓do.
15  Pt:   O↑kay,
16  SiL:  O↑kay,
17  MD:   I do palliative medicine, ↓which is kind of newer sp↑ecialty in
18        medicine?
19  SiL:  O↑kay,
20  MD:   Have you ever heard of it:, (0.4)
21  SiL:  ↑Sure?
22  MD:   Have you heard of that ↑before?
23  SiL:  Sure,
```

24 MD: You ↑have?
25 Pt: Sure.

The physician's design for the first portion of this interaction has had positive rapport-building results, which we can see reinforced in the exchanges above, though we are not able to account for gaze direction and eye contact in lines 17–23. The evolving self-identification among the family members in lines 3–11 – from "*his* daughter" to "*the* wife" and then to "*the* spouse" – expresses an increasing level of depersonalized abstraction that, we believe, reveals not a resistance to the clinician's (self-)presentation, but rather an accommodation of it. By presenting the family as an orderly, typical, memorable abstraction, the family engage in a profound gesture of accommodation to this stranger, recycling templates of self-representations they have learned over multiple hospital visits together. As a family facing the protracted suffering of one of its members, this kind of self-presentation as "the wife", for instance, is one of the ways patients' families affirmatively inscribe themselves into the institutional needs of the clinicians they interact with (see also Antaki 2011a; Atkinson 1995; Barton 2004; Barton 2015; Barton et al. 2005; Herndl and Nahrwold 2000; Sarangi and Roberts 1999). We will see in conversation 2.2 below a situation in which family members, with evident good reason, do not offer such an autoethnographic accommodation through abstraction (Agar 1996 [1980]).

Subsequent to the clinician's self-humbling gesture in line 2 above, he switches in line 14 from affiliative, pronominal *we*-subject to the active vocational anchoring "what I do," accompanied by strong declarative intonation, emphatically highlighting not the "I" but the "do" (see Couper-Kuhlen 2012a). Noteworthy is that in this turn he does not introduce Palliative Care itself, nor present himself as a *potential* group-level practitioner of it, but as someone who *does certain things*, regardless of disciplinary constraints or of his prospective intention to *do those things* in this patient's particular situation.

In subtle ways, the physician is also updating the rhetorical gravitas of the classic mid-20th-century expert model of hospital doctor identity. Continuing, he reframes "what I do" (expert activity, line 14 above) into "what I [...] get asked to do" (vocation/calling):

1 MD: ↑Okay(.)- Um (1.0) ↑<What I typically> get asked to do here in the <u>hospital</u>
2   is kind of two things. (.) <One i:s> ah often come by to help people ↓with
3   whatever symptom's bo↓thering ↓them.
4 Pt: Okay,
5 MD: ↑Most often it's <u>pain.</u>

 5 SiL: Okay,
 6 MD: Constipation, <u>nau:</u>sea, (1.0) (cough)) <u>depression</u>, ↑you name it,=If it's
 7   bothering ↓you (.) my <u>job</u> is to try and help- ↑make them feel better.
 8 Pt: ↑Okay.
 9 MD: ↑Okay, the other <u>thing</u> I-[thank you   ]
10   ((chairs moving))
11 Uk: [((whispered))]
12 MD: >↑Do you want a chair?<
13 SiL: No, I'm ↑good, thank you.
14 MD: ↑>You're good?<Yeah, okay.
15 SiL: Yeah.

By describing what he "typically" does, and what he passively "gets asked to do", rather than what he is "here for", the physician is able to establish a kind of preliminary protective boundary between him (and what he represents) and the patient/ family, who are invited to view and understand this physician at a safe distance as *someone with a vocation* – as opposed to as someone who has come to do something *to us*, or someone with a self-referential *profession* or self-serving *agenda* (on the interactional structure of invitations generally, see Davidson 1984). As the family members and patient have continued thus far to respond to the physician's presentation primarily with one-word assent tokens ("Yeah," "Okay," and "Sure") and with abiding though interrogative intonation, their polite but noncommittal stances suggest that the physician's cautious bearing is still called for.

The clinician's presentation of Palliative Care, by way of a classic expert vocational model and its various *I/we* deictic formulations, continues:

 1 MD: ↑Oh so sorry- ((chairs moving)) ↑>The other <u>thing</u> that we often get asked
 2   to do< is to kind of <sit <u>dow:</u>n, ↓um,> and help <u>people</u> ↑kind of under-
 3   stand ↑everythi:ng we find (0.8) with the <u>medicines</u> and the testing and
 4   all those things in the <u>hospital</u> ↓or (.) you know even before coming into
 5   the ↓hospital= ↑And understand what does that really mean for ↑you
 6   (.) And what are your ↑options (.) in terms ↓of, kind of next ↓steps=↑And
 7   where do we go from ↓here
 8 Pt: ↑Okay.
 9 MD: My understanding <u>is</u> (.) ↑we're here mostly for that second ↓part=↑kind of
10   reviewing <u>everything</u>, >looking at <u>options</u><(.) ↓Um (0.8) does that sound
11   about ↑right?
12 Dt: Yes.
13 Sp: Mm-hmm.
14 SiL: Yeah.

15 MD: Okay.=↑Any questions for <u>me</u> before we be↓gin. (2.2)
16 Pt: ↑I'm going to be a silent <u>part</u>ner here, so, you folks-
17 RN: ↑Not yet.
18 Dt: ↑[Not yet.   ] hh ((laughter))
19 SiL: ↑[You've got to keep going-]
20 MD: ↑I'll, I'll ask that question of↓ten.
21 Pt: Okay.
22 MD: ↑So then let me ask ↓<u>you</u> (.) what is your under<u>standing</u> of kind of
23   ↓where things are with your disease or what's going on,
24 Pt: Well (.) it's ↑obviously <u>termi</u>↓nal (0.8) Um, we don't have a <u>time</u>frame.
25   =<It:'s relatively short> (.) lifespan available to me (.)

In this section, common clinician-initiated metaphors from Palliative Care discourse first make their appearance, such as "next steps" and "options" (see Appleton and Flynn 2014). But the physician phrases his invitation for a confirmatory response in line 10–11 in a specific way – not as "does that sound good," but "does that sound about right?" This is a bid not for an affirmative evaluation of what he has presented to them just then, but for a confirmation (or correction) of an existing reality they have witnessed, independent of the physician, with its own history of development. The patient's prospective need for a conversation about "next steps" is elicited not by way of persuasion and proposition on the clinician's part, but with recourse to family members' ongoing reflections. In general, the physician develops a mixed-vernacular approach, using short phrases like "what I do", "here to talk", "know who's who", "ever heard of it?", "you name it", "make it feel better" – usually followed by some form of bid for confirmation from the group (Gardner 2001).

It is only after deploying each of these three complex interactional moves – deictic shifts, mixed vernacularity, and social joining through status recognition and project concession – that the physician asks for any questions from the group "before we begin." Here, the physician re-issues his previous announcement from line 10 (on page 48) that "we" are "here to talk", only proceeding to do so after he has received confirmation that such talking is indeed "okay," in lines 17–18 above. Such metadiscursive gestures, i.e. explicit reflections about the act of interacting through talk, continue to emerge, as the physician announces in line 20 above that "I'll ask that question often." Here, he is bridging the current pre-conversation to the incipient conversation, by way of a promise that there will be some predictable regularity in its features and structure. He has already taken authoritative responsibility for the conduct of the conversation through the promise "I'll ask" and through descriptions of predictability "what I do." Through this combination of metadiscursive and promissory features, the physician's project is not only "introducing Palliative Care" as such but, more crucially, introducing himself as a *kind of* speaker and as a responsible representative of a certain kind of conversation. These three sections above show the complex social initiation of a clinician, through the negotiation and elaboration of face, role, credentials, entitlement, self-restraint, ground rules, and procedural disclosure. And yet, none of the clinician talk comes across as prolix, coercive, or overly self-conscious.

The patient appears to have received the clinician's initial project and strategy well, considering it legitimate enough to respond to in kind with forthright, informative concision – which is of course only one potential way to confer legitimacy on an interlocutor. As we noted above, lines 6–7 on the top of page 51 contain a kind of jump-shift, in which the patient takes the clinician's formulaic "what is your understanding" question and immediately raises the stakes from understanding to prognosis (Butow et al. 2002). He uses a particular kind of language to do this, namely the speech genre of business logistics: "relatively short timeframe" and "available to me", which corresponds co-stylistically to the casual but serviceable business vernacular of the physician in lines 6–7 on the top of page 51. A telling difference emerges stylistically between them in lines 22–25 above, when the clinician asks the patient to describe "*kind of* where things are with your disease" (on vagueness and indirection, see Lerner 2011; on 'doing neutrality, see Clayman 1998). The patient gently rebukes the physician's roundabout formulation with the unhesitating response, "Well it's obviously terminal." Here, the patient refers to his disease as an "it", where the clinician uses "your" twice to ascribe possession to the patient's "understanding" and "disease," though this possessive ascription is not emphasized prosodically (Morgan 2010).

The generic project of "re-presenting Palliative Care" tends, perhaps because of its conversation-initial position, to be a monologic one that disprefers unprompted interruption. We note that the patient in line 16 above symbolically indexes, claims, and reframes this asymmetry of physician-initiated topic-introduction talk, positioning himself preemptively as "[I'm going to be] the silent partner." The metaphor of the silent partner illustrates some features of the Palliative Care consultation generally, while also reinforcing some of the status-maintenance goals the patient had initiated earlier on. A silent partner in a business accepts self-marginalization, and yet retains rights to centrality as an investor or guarantor. This is only the first of scores of instances in this book where a seriously-ill patient notices and illustrates some of the ironies of power and powerlessness constituting his overall position within hospital discourse and within the currently emerging interactional relations (Back et al. 2009; Bartels et al. 2016; see also Jefferson 1989; Kulick 2005). In line 24, the patient nonetheless casts off this "silent" position, volunteering a summary of how he understands the current state of his illness. Thus, he is able to style himself both marginal and simultaneously authoritative in the current social constellation.

This conversation is one that Palliative Care clinicians would often regard as having the makings of a successful decisional consultation around *goals-of-care*, because the participants were able to achieve agreement and mutual recognition about disease prognosis, allowing the conversation then to move toward quality-of-life-based decision-making. Given that this person was physiologically able to live only 34 more days past this consultation, accomplishing mutual acknowledgement around a prognosis in this interaction was crucial for envisioning goals of care for the upcoming weeks. The clinician's ability to negotiate the social joining process, to design his own framework for legitimation and ratification by the group, to announce and structure what it meant to be "here to talk", and his willingness to translate between multiple vernaculars each contributed to this success.

*For further examples of **social joining**, see conversations 3.1, 5.4. For **meta-discursive markers**, see 8.1, 9.2., 5.1, 5.3. For patients' bid for **status recognition**, see 3.5, 8.1, 5.3, 2.3, 10.7, 5.4. For idioms and metaphors of **business negotiation**, see 10.3, 6.4. For instances of discord between **frankness and indirection**, see 4.5, 6.1–2, 7.3, 8.3, 8.5, 9.2, 10.12.*

2.2 Tell me what you need

The successful tactics and orientations evident in conversation 2.1 are thrown into deep relief when contrasted with the next conversation, where the re-presentation of Palliative Care quickly encounters umbrage from the patient and family who, quite rationally, hold the consulting clinician responsible for broader logistical problems they've experienced in the hospital setting thus far. In our analysis of the following conversation, we ask:

1) What are the techniques and premises by which patients (implicitly or explicitly) resist interaction with a Palliative Care clinician, and what preexisting and emerging circumstances prompt them to do so?

2) How does a Palliative Care clinician come across, when persisting nonetheless in her attempts to repair, or salvage, the occasion to re-present Palliative Care, when met with contestation and refusal? (see Couper-Kuhlen 1992; Curl 2005; Drew 1997; Egbert 2004; see also Jefferson 1974)?

3) What happens when family members and patients attempt to elicit specific information from Palliative Care clinicians that is beyond the scope of their roles as they've presented them?

4) Under what circumstances may it be imprudent to initiate or continue a consultation?
5) How do phenomena of discordance in Palliative Care conversations intersect with gendered, religious, and racialized features of interaction?

The hospitalized person in the following conversation self-identifies as a 75-year-old Black woman and as financially secure, reporting Associate's-level education and Christian religious affiliation. She has been diagnosed with a stage-four lung cancer. She believes she is "likely" to live for a year, while her clinician-rated survival prognosis at the time of the following consultation was two weeks to three months, thus indicating strong prognostic discordance between patient and clinician. In fact, she continued to live for 123 days after this consultation: longer than clinicians expected, but shorter than she herself expected at the time of consultation. The patient ranks her end-of-life goals as "comfort over longevity," and she rates her "global" quality-of-life over the previous two days as a six out of ten. The following portion of talk occurred during the first visit of the Palliative Care team. The clinician speaking in this consultation is a Palliative Care nurse practitioner.

1 Pt: .hh Sorry .hh
2 NP: ↑It's okay (.) ↑We're with the <u>Pal</u>↑liative Care Team. (0.5)
3 Pt: ↑I'm so sick of you ↑<u>people</u> hh((laughter))
4 NP: What's ↑wrong?
5 Pt: What do ↑<u>you</u> want. (1.0)
6 NP: Do you- is ↑now not a good ↑<u>ti:me</u>?
7 Pt: Uh tell me what you ↓need. (0.8)
8 NP: hh hh (0.2) Well ↑tell me who's here with ↑<u>you</u>.
9 Dt: We're her <u>children</u>.=We're her <u>daughters</u>,
10 NP: ↑Hi,
11 Dt: Hi,

In the opening sequence of this conversation, two primary speakers (clinician and patient) appear to 'get off on the wrong foot.' They competitively ignore one another's questions or resist the premises upon which they are asked, resulting in an overt conversational tenor of mistrust, misfire, and incredulousness. Though the patient is perhaps bolder in waving off the clinician's questions about "what's wrong" and whether it is "not a good time", the clinician is equally unwilling to grant the premise that she herself is here needing something. Indeed, the nurse practitioner's response "What's wrong?" to the patient's immediately preceding utterance "I'm so sick of you people" appears to be a strategic misinterpretation. It attributes the patient's frustration to something physiologically "wrong" (i.e., something ailing the patient) rather than, perhaps, "wrong" with the institutional order, including the "you people" the patient has just invoked.

Clearly, the participants in this conversation did not enjoy the underlying circumstances of good faith and expediency salient in conversation 2.1, where the physician was able, relatively easily and quickly, to present a socially credible version of the "re-presenting Palliative Care" project, to which the family members were willing to grant provisional legitimacy. Here in conversation 2.2, in line 3, the patient is poised to preempt any pre-designed presentational strategy structuring the conversation, "wrong-footing" the nurse practitioner (Goffman 1979) with the bald on-record positive face threat "I'm so sick of you people," and then quickly laughing in an ostensively friendly way so as to redress and redistribute face. The clinician tries to repair with "What's wrong?" and "Is now not a good time?", but the patient dismisses these disingenuously informational elicitations with the abidingly impatient non-sequitur "Tell me what you need." This idiomatically cordial demand again threatens the nurse practitioner's positive face, by placing her in the position of someone who *needs something* but will not 'come out with it.'

Further on, the patient also threatens the nurse practitioner's negative face by prompting her to disclose what exactly she has planned for the incipient consultation (see line 5 and 9 below). The patient is interested in actions, rather than words, and wishes to compel the nurse practitioner to get down to the business of medical treatment, if indeed she has any such business to get down to. This is thus a 'put your cards out on the table' situation.

With seriously-ill people, we find it sometimes helps to understand hospital-based interactions through symbolic relations of home and hospitality, particularly given that patients' hospital rooms may be, and are often, the last experience of home they have the ability to lay claim to. The emerging dynamics in this conversation make particular sense when viewed as the appropriate relations between a person at home minding their own business and an unwelcome, pestering stranger. By framing herself as a person who can fulfill others' needs (in line 7 above), including those of the clinician, the patient additionally assigns to herself the metaphorical status of a service-and-information-provider who is able, if not yet quite willing, to accommodate the needs of unscheduled outsiders, a characterization that is contrasted, already by line 8, with a resulting impression of the clinician as a not entirely forthcoming and honest needer.

Thus far, the patient has preemptively gotten off a highly off-putting face threat "sick of you people," redressing it only by *doing* friendly laughter in line 3 (see Glenn 1989; Glenn 1995; Haakana 2001; Haakana 2002). Pragmatic failure is thus the emerging interactional idiom. In contrast also to conversation 2.1, where family members were inclined to inscribe themselves into a neutral map of family relations germane to the interpretive order of the hospital staff, no such self-ironizing, self-alienating gesture of accommodation is evident here. The patient's daughter adopts a much more personalized, emphatic, and protective stance about family relations, indicating that she feels drawn to anticipate adversarial relations requiring defensive tactics and social buffering. Already within four turns at talk, in the course of which three instances of unrepaired pragmatic failure have ensued, these dynamics of mutual nonaccommodation have established themselves somewhat firmly.

1 NP: Um (0.8) so ↑I am with the pal↑liative care ↓team.
2 Pt: Uh huh.=Uh huh.
3 NP: Um ↑<and they asked us to> come and help with some of your ↑symptoms.
4 (1.0)
5 Pt: What symptoms. (.) ↓can you deal ↓with
6 NP: ↑Some shortness of breath I heard you were having. (0.8)
7 Pt: Palliative care do:es (0.8) ↑medical? (0.8)
8 NP: Mm-hmm,
9 Pt: Okay.=What are you going to ↓do. (1.0)
10 NP: ↑So (.) let- well ((coughing)) let me tell you what- what we- (0.5) what we
11 ↑do do ↓ okay?
12 Pt: Okay.

Here, the idiom of disorientation and nonrecognition continues, with competing footings as to whether the current order of business is discussing *being* something (i.e. being a member of the Palliative Care team), doing something *now* (alleviating symptoms), or doing something *later* (planning to alleviate symptoms), etc. The patient appears to be aware that the clinician wishes to enumerate the features of the specialty or institutional resource she represents, and is disinclined to permit her to do so unimpeded. Furthermore, the patient seems intent on expediting the talk toward action, dismissing the inherent value of talk or presentation as an end in itself, or as a useful resource for clinical purposes. For her part, the clinician has framed her role similarly as had the physician in conversation 2.1 as "with the palliative care team," but does not qualify it further as a collective omnipresence so much as a delegating body, a "they" that "asked us to come." This image of provenance around the referral does little to allay the patient's dismay.

The patient's earnest but elliptical question in line 6 above, "Palliative Care does medical?", deserves some specific attention, especially given her nearly second-long pause before "medical." Her proposed distinction of "medical" (vs. non-medical) seems poised to delimit what she had previously imagined Palliative

Care to be: a form of hospital-based social work or social service with little clinical impact. In lines 9–10, there emerges a tension between the patient's revised characterization of Palliative Care as a latent battery of enumerable medical capabilities the patient might avail herself of as needed and what the clinician wishes for it to be acknowledged as: a responsive, discerning specialty capable of addressing the symptoms "I heard you've been having." The next section of the talk, the re-presentation of Palliative Care proper, indeed shows some similarities on the thematic level with that in conversation 2.1 above.

1	NP:	↑S:o there's a couple of different <u>parts</u> to what we <u>do:</u>.=The the <u>first</u> thing
2		is-the ↑first part of what we <u>do</u> is helping with symp<u>toms</u> ↑<u>short</u>ness
3		of <u>breath</u> (.) <u>pain</u>, (0.8) um (.) consti↑pa<u>tion</u> feeling <u>anx</u>ious (.) feeling
4		<u>depressed</u> ↓anything like <u>that</u> ↑>We're very good at getting those <u>things</u><
5		under con<u>trol</u> (0.5) so that ↑you (.) can do the things that <u>you</u> ↑want to ↓do.
6		(0.8) ↑The <u>second</u> part of <what we <u>do</u> is t:o> (0.2) get more ↑<u>information</u>
7		about your medical issues? and ↑to answer ques<u>tions</u> that you <u>have</u> ↑if- if
8		there are decisions that need to be ↑made? ((coughing)) ↑And to help you
9		figure out what the <u>best</u> <u>thing</u> is for <u>you</u> ↓in your situa↓tion. ((clearing of
10		throat)) And then the ↑<u>third</u> <u>part</u> (.) of what we do (.) ↓because we're very
11		good at the <u>symptoms</u> and <u>helping</u> with difficult deci↓sions is we do some
12		end of life ↓care. (0.8) That's <u>not</u> why we're here to see ↑<u>you</u> to↓day (0.8)
13		but they ↑asked us to come and help with some <u>symp</u>toms and see if we
14		could be: of <u>support</u> to you and your family (0.5) .hh as deci↓sions need to
15		be ↓made. (2.8) Do you have any ques↑tions about that? (0.8)
16	Pt:	<u>No</u> (.) Uh let me- let me tell ↓<u>you</u>.
17	NP:	↑Okay.
18	Pt:	I ↑<u>figured</u> at this ↑point (0.8) ( ) (1.0) be↓cause I have not heard from
19		On<u>co</u>logy from <u>doc</u>tors saying (0.2) where you ↑are ↓now.

In line 13–15, at the end of the uninterrupted multipart presentation of Palliative Care, the clinician uses passive and somewhat euphemistic phrases: "being of support to you and your family as decisions need to be made." It is the latter clause in this sentence that seems to participate in a euphemistic genre that trades on vagary and nontransparency as to who makes what decisions. As we can see, then, conversations 2.1 and 2.2 represent a spectrum of options for clinicians during initial consultations. The designs of social joining, deictic modulation, metalinguistic framing, and mixed vernacularity, so smoothly available to the physician in 2.1 have become less viable in 2.2.

In an intriguing inversion of the self-presentation strategies in 2.1, the patient in 2.2 demands somewhat exasperatedly of the clinician that she say clearly "what you're gonna do," at which point the clinician balks and redirects away from this idiom of intention towards a resource that the physician in 2.1 had found quite useful: characterizing typical Palliative Care activities instead, and giving an account of "what we *do* do." But whereas in 2.1 this had been a genial and strategically attuned selection, here it appears to be a dodge into insincerity. The patient registers this in line 16, then, as the third instance so far in which the clinician has dodged her (the patient's) own direct question or request, giving evidence for the patient's emerging project of disqualifying the clinician as cagey, ulterior, and equivocal. Having her customary resources undermined in this way, the clinician then seems to rush the "introducing Palliative Care" project, moving from clause to clause without pausing for confirmation, lest the patient find means to wrong-foot her further.

Patiently waiting for the clinician to finish her presentation, the patient then deflects a "Do you have any questions about that" volley with a resolute "No, let me tell *you*," in line 16. What the patient wishes to "tell you" remains for the moment ambiguous and open; telling may be understood in this moment as an informational act and also as an act of status, that of someone who has the authority to "tell." As with conversation 2.1, the patient asserts autonomy and status, but here in 2.2 the assertion of that status is contentious rather than convivial. "Telling" allows the patient to take up the symbolic position of dictation and conveyance, reversing what she treats as an illegitimate knowledge-power relation. By now, it is clear that at least the first four of the five complicating circumstances detailed in the introduction to this chapter are in play: uncertainty about the provenance of the referral, patient ambivalence, discipline fatigue, and (referring) clinician ambiguity. In line 19, it becomes clear that much of the patient's disinterest is not directed toward Palliative Care itself, but rather towards its unexpected insertion into the overall sequence of rounding among other urgently expected specialists, here an oncologist who has not yet made a vaguely scheduled appearance.

Patients' and families' interactions with oncologists and other curative specialties constitute a major recurring topic in many Palliative Care conversations, and patients express, and highly prioritize, the value of clear demonstration of effective information-sharing between Palliative Care and oncology. Perception on the patient's or family's part that adequate information-sharing has not yet taken place can scuttle a successful Palliative Care consultation already in its introductory moments.

Though this conversation does not (in or beyond the transcribed portions) thematize race and ethnicity in any explicit way, it is nonetheless relevant that Black patients referred for Palliative Care (such as this woman) have often been subject to a meaningfully different history of patienthood and curative discourse than white patients have. "In African-American communities," suggests Steven

Wakefield, effectively reaching communities often "means working to replace a legacy of distrust – rooted in the Tuskegee syphilis experiment" (Motin Goff 2005). Black patients referred for Palliative Care consultations, particularly by or with non-Black clinicians, may bring to the interaction rational forms of historical suspicion that implicitly reference previous clinical generations' unwillingness to pursue aggressive treatments for Black patients or, in the Tuskegee experiments of 1932–1972, willingness to expose Black patients to life-threatening viruses in ways that perpetuated ongoing anti-Black racism. Such interactions are always historical in some underlying way, and race, gender, and religious identity point to some of the historical vectors of privilege and peril that shape these consultations.

For further **metaphors of hospitality and home-making**, see 4.3. For patients' strategies for **undermining clinicians' agendas**, see 9.2, 8.5, 8.2, 8.1, 7.3. For the **interactional saliency of gender and race**, see 5.3, 5.2.

2.3 The whole role and all that

One way to re-present Palliative Care in an initial consultation is to not do so at all, or to represent the field and its potential offerings elliptically or tersely. In the following conversation, we are interested in exploring what it sounds like when a clinician sees fit to truncate or forego the re-presentation of Palliative Care in a consultation altogether, having become convinced that the patient or family already grasps what it is and needs no review. We ask:
1. How does such a circumstance emerge, and on what basis has a clinician assessed this rationale for a truncated introduction of Palliative Care?
2. What phenomena of mutual confirmation take place when a shared yet unspecified referent "Palliative Care" is being mobilized by participants, who see fit to believe they share a mutual understanding, or wish to sidestep the event of presentation altogether?
3. When is a truncated re-presentation prudent, and for what reasons?

The patient in this conversation self-identifies as a 62-year-old white man and as financially insecure, reporting high-school-level education and Christian religious affiliation. He has been diagnosed with a stage-four esophageal cancer. He believes he is "very likely" to live for a year, while his clinician-rated survival prognosis at the time of the following consultation is three to six months. In fact, he continued to live for 39 days after this consultation, i.e., shorter than both he and the clinical team expected at the time of consultation. The patient ranks his end-of-life goals as moderately "comfort over longevity," and he rates his "global" quality-of-life over the previous two days as a nine out of ten. The following portion of talk occurred during the first visit of the Palliative Care team. The clinician speaking is an internal medicine resident doing a two-week rotation on the Palliative Care service.

1 Res: ↑Um (0.2) did, =did the: ↑<u>onc</u>ology team tell you- tell you guys about (0.5)
2   Palliative Care and [<what we <u>do</u> and all that?>]
3 FM1:   [↑Oh he's very fam<u>il</u>iar=]
4 FM2: =↑He's fa [miliar. °Yeah.°]
5 Res: [>↑Okay=↑So, so] you've seen< Palliative Care in the <u>pas:t</u>?
6 Sp: ↑Yes.

Here, the clinician (who is not trained in Palliative Care but is currently a resident on a two-week training with the Palliative Care service), asks the patient's family to confirm that they know "what we do and all that". The two family members' confirmatory response is "he's very familiar" – a predicate adjective that tends to come with a predicate object, such as "familiar with Palliative Care", "familiar with what you do", or simply "familiar with it" etc., but any such object is elided in both family members' latched responses in lines 3–4. In going with this generally dispreferred or truncated (but emphatic) formulation "he's very familiar", both responding family members may be interactionally favoring ambiguity at this turn. They do not intuitively wish to indicate what exactly their loved one, the patient, is familiar with. This could be an assertion of general hospital know-how, and not a particular understanding of the specialty of Palliative Care. Or, it may be a polite resistance to the incipience of the presentation itself, for any number of reasons.

Their response also seems an important *implicature* (by way of their violating the maxims of Quality (Grice 1975), in addition to Manner with the dispreferred usage of "familiar", as noted above), in the sense that the family members are obviously not answering the clinician's question – whether "oncology" told them what Palliative Care was. The clinician did relatively little to push for clarification about the answer to his question, or to take cues from the complex implicature at hand. It is further noteworthy that the clinician (an internist in training) appears to assume that "oncology's" imagined explanation of Palliative Care is reliable on its face, and he allows it to stand as a referential basis for their further volleys of confirmation. "See[ing] Palliative Care" in line 5 is an ambiguous referent too, as the clinician takes as given that the patient and family can and will distinguish in this interaction between palliative modalities as they may be expressed and practiced by oncologists (in past visits) and direct care from a Palliative Care physician or PC nurse practitioner. These are ambiguities that, collectively, ensure a very loose shared repertoire of imagined references between the clinician and family, which continues as follows:

1 Res: ↑Okay, so you know the whole <u>role</u>: and all ↓that.
2 Pt: °[↓Mm-hmm].°
3 Sp: °[Right].°
4 Res: They <u>more</u> focus just on: like: (0.4) <u>symp</u>tom management >and that kind
5   of [↓thing.]<
6 Sp: [↓Right]
7 Res: >So any,< (0.5) any symptoms of: <u>discomfort</u> <you're ↓having we can
8   con<u>trol</u>: and >(.)[what↓ever.]
9 Sp: [Right.]
10 Pt: [↓Right=]
11 Res: [Okay=]
12 Sp: [=Yes]

The clinician's gloss of the specialty of Palliative Care in lines 4–5 is arguably not quite an adequate portrayal, in that it relies on "symptom management" as a synecdoche for a number of the discipline's further clinical functions, as elaborated in conversations 2.1 and 2.2. The nominalized institutional abstraction "symptom management" – rather than for example "how we deal with symptoms' – increases this potential for misunderstanding. The clinician does go the extra step of providing a description of what "symptom management" means, but does not provide examples of the kind of "discomfort" Palliative Care can address, as conversations 2.1 and 2.2 do.

This instance of "re-presenting Palliative Care" contrasts with the previous two, in the sense that the clinician intuitively sees fit to truncate the introduction on the apparent basis of expediency and an imagined shared referent. We notice that there are multiple additional discursive forces at work in this conversation, including the *absent* oncology team, whose previous contributions serve as the apparent catalyst for foregoing the presentational project. As noted above, when asked whether the oncology team had "told you guys about palliative care and what we do and all that," the family member responds with "He's very familiar." We find that this response functions primarily as a bid for status acknowledgement on the patient's behalf, and not as a substantive claim or confirmation about the patient's knowledge as such. The clinician nonetheless takes this response as referential rather than performative, and his interpretive choice prompts a sequence in which the participants co-construct a shared referent of "Palliative Care" that, it is assumed, can then be acted upon without ambiguity. The clinician chooses to *speed through* the "introducing Palliative Care" project, pivoting to various referential items that are formulated in diminutive and circumscribed terms ("and all that", "whatever", etc.). Having established that the patient and spouse have "seen Palliative Care in the past" the clinician deduces that "you know the whole role and all that, that they're, that they more focus just on, like, symptom management and that kinda thing." Interestingly, the clinician's deictic framing of Palliative Care shifts from "they" in "they focus on" to "we" in "we can control"; this suggests the clinician favors identification with active clinical interventions more than with observational and interpretive functions, such as "focusing".

Relieved to see confirmative assertions in the form of the patient and patient's spouse's "He's very familiar" and "Right, right", the clinician sees fit to assume a truncated shared understanding of what Palliative Care is, even though "symptom management," referred to here in the nominalized short-hand, is only one component of the discipline, and does not have an easily intuitive relationship with the other components. It is perhaps the case that the clinician sees this imagined shared knowledge as a source of rapport-building between them, whereas an exploratory reintroduction of Palliative Care might undermine that rapport momentum.

For further examples of **truncated explanations**, *see 9.3, 3.3, 6.3. For* **deictic disidentifications and identifications**, *see 2.5. For patients' strategies for* **establishing status through epistemic stance**, *see 3.5, 8.1, 5.3, 10.7, 5.4. For other cases with* **medical students and residents**, *see 8.1, 4.5.*

2.4 A fancy word

Similar to 2.3, the following conversation exhibits features that suggest the clinician is not entirely comfortable presenting Palliative Care directly, pivoting either to presumed shared understandings or taking recourse to another discourse, namely that of "supportive care." We are therefore interested here in the question:

1. How do clinicians seek to "translate" official or semi-official definitions of Palliative Care into terms they feel, spontaneously or otherwise, better fit the needs of the clinical setting?

The patient in the following conversation self-identifies as a 67-year-old white man and as financially secure, reporting middle-school-level education and Christian religious affiliation. He has been diagnosed with a stage-four sarcoma, i.e., a soft-tissue tumor. He believes he is "very likely" to live for a year, and his clinician-rated survival prognosis at the time of the following consultation is more than six months. In fact, he continued living beyond the six-month follow-up period of the study, which means both clinician and patient expectations at the time of consultation were accurate. The patient strongly ranks his end-of-life goals as "comfort over longevity," and he rates his "global" quality-of-life over the previous two days – i.e., physical, emotional, social, spiritual, and financial quality – as a five out of ten. The following portion of talk occurred during the first visit of the Palliative Care team. The clinician speaking in the conversation is a Palliative Care physician.

```
 1  MD:  Um: and um =well so in terms of who we are and I may have-
 2  Pt:   Mm-hmm?
 3  MD:  talked a bit about this but (.) um: we're Palliative ↑Care (.) and we were (.)
 4        asked by the oncology team to come and- and help out with your your pain
 5        management. ↑Palliative Care is kind of of- a fancy wor:d um =but a bet-
 6        better word for it might be ↑supportive care because we support people
 7        and families (.) who have serious ill↑ness? in lots of different ways.=And
 8        one of the big-the ↑big ways >very common ways that we help< people
 9        is with ↑symptom management very difficult to (.) control symptoms as-
10        with like your- (0.5) your pain.
11  Pt:   >Yep.<
12  MD:  Nausea >shortness of breath <there's lots of different symptoms,
13  Pt:   >Uh huh.<
```

In this exchange, the physician presents "Palliative Care" negatively, in both the differential and the evaluative sense of the word negative. He casts off *palliative* in line 5 as a "fancy word" for something, for which a "better" word would be *supportive* care. Indeed, as we noted in the introductory chapter, a predominant discourse of "supportive care" does exist in literature and health care policy, particularly in Australia, where the National Institute for Health and Care Excellence defines supportive care as: "helping the patient to maximise the benefits of treatment and to live as well as possible with the effects of the disease" (NICE 2004: 18). This definition champions a philosophy or mode of care that can be pursued by multiple branches of medicine, not just Palliative Care itself, an advocacy stance we might refer to as a 'majoritizing' strategy. To be sure, the hospice and palliative care *movements* did not abate with the establishment of a board-certified PC medical specialty, and clinicians such as the physician in this conversation find ways to advocate for a broader agenda of palliative modalities throughout the hospital setting. Patients may however find "supportive care" to be an unnecessarily redundant and therefore ambiguous label; one might ask, for instance, should not all care be "supportive" in some meaningful way?

The physician's presentation continues:

```
1   MD:   <Um people have ↑problems with and- and (.) that's one of our areas of
2         expertise: =Um: (.) another um =area that we help with is ↑information
3         sharing?=Um folks with serious illness u- =often have a ↑lo:t of information
4         they need to: (.) to get to understand- make sense of and- and uh we help
5         with communications because that information doesn't ↑always get to
6         °↓you° um in a way that is meaningful to you =So (.) we help with that? >We
7         also help with< um (0.5) uh- (0.5) de↑cision making in terms of- uh treatment
8         options =Because sometimes that can get really ↓complicated=We help with
9         that we help with um coordination of care=°That can get really complicated
10        sometimes° too=↑So >we help them with lots and lots of different °things.°<
11  Pt:   Mm-hmm.
12  MD:   But the main (.) a main ↑way we've been asked to (.) come help you with
13        today is is for ↓management of °this pain,° Um: (.) and (0.8) I understand
14        that ↑it's-it's ↑fairly recent where the pain has been like really trouble↓some
15        for you=like you've ↑had it in the past but it's not been really a: a big deal.
16  Pt:   Mm-hmm,
17  MD:   ↑When did it start really becoming a (.) you know a ↑burden to you?
18  Pt:   Uh: (2.2) about three ↑weeks ago?
19  MD:   Uh huh.
20  Pt:   I:t's ↑fairly new to me ↑too?
```

Here, again, "supportive care" is enumerated as including symptom management, information management, decision-making, and coordination-of-care. These are each introduced as nominalized items and then justified through typical causal circumstances and optimal outcomes in each instance. Information management in Palliative Care is that feature of care which ensures that information "gets to you in a way that is meaningful to you." Listening politely through this definition during which the physician holds the floor through self-latching at most TRPs (turn-relevance places), the patient responds intermittently with acknowledgement tokens of "mm-hmm," which are audibly constrained by the sensations of pain, which had prompted the oncology team to make the Palliative Care referral.

At the beginning of the exchange, the physician inquires about when the sarcoma was diagnosed, then proceeds into a description of "who we are." The most predominant features of this style of re-presentation are then a) its majoritizing gesture of associating Palliative Care as a specialty with broader, ubiquitous palliative and hospice-related practices throughout health care landscapes and b) the deliberate and explicit endeavor to effectively translate the field and its self-understandings into terms that are less "fancy" and more "meaningful" to the patient and family.

*For further examples of **majoritizing stances on Palliative Care**, see 2.5. For **emphasis on what is meaningful to patients**, see 4.4, 7.4. For **information sharing**, see 5.3, 9.3, 9.5. For **vernacular translations of clinical concepts**, see 3.5, 7.5, 6.1–2, 6.5, 2.1, 6.4, 7.3.*

2.5 I think that's actually everybody

In conversation 2.4, we saw a physician set aside the official board-certified designation "Palliative Care," in favor of a description that accommodates, under the label of "supportive care," a spectrum of related practices throughout the hospital setting. In the next conversation, we see a further instance of a majoritizing portrayal, in which a Palliative Care clinician depicts her specialty in an expansive way that accentuates its universal relevance throughout the hospital, thereby gaining interactional legitimacy in various ways.

The patient in the following conversation self-identifies as a 55-year-old white woman and as financially secure, reporting Associate's-level education and Christian religious affiliation. She has been diagnosed with a stage-four breast cancer. She believes she is "very likely" to live for a year, while her clinician-rated survival prognosis at the time of the following consultation is two weeks to three months. In fact, she lived five days beyond this consultation, i.e., drastically shorter than both she and the Palliative Care clinicians expected. The patient strongly ranks her end-of-life goals as "comfort over longevity," and she rates her "global" quality-of-life over the previous two days – i.e., physical, emotional, social, spiritual, and financial quality – at a five out of ten. The following portion of talk occurred during the first visit of the Palliative Care team. The clinician is a Palliative Care nurse practitioner.

1	NP:	Um: (.) He =I (.) have a lot of respect for, for him=.hhh um (1.2) so from
2		Palliative Care, what usually happens is: one of uh=the >°nurse
3		practitio↓ners°< usually comes °first and we just sort of° gather ↓information.
4	Sp:	>Okay.<
5	NP:	I work with an attending <u>physician</u>,
6	Sp:	Okay.
7	NP:	Um: and (.) he will ↑probably? come by to↑morrow.
8	Sp:	Okay.
9	NP:	°If that's all right.°
10	Sp:	Yeah.
11	NP:	I don't think there's any <u>urgency</u>?
12	Sp:	[Yeah.]

13 NP: [I don't know] if you sense that,=Um- and if you do, I can
14   simpl[y call him.]
15 Sp: [↑No, I don't] any more=that seemed to be- (0.8) you know=right at
16   the beginning there was (.) they were talking about like ↓discharge >°after
17   the (.) and I got really upset about that because it's-°<
18 NP: [Scary.]
19 Sp: [So ob]viously, not. ↑not what °should have happened° ( ) =But that's
20   all o↓ver.

As with conversations 2.1–2 and 2.4, the clinician begins to describe Palliative Care
here as a typical and predictable set of visits and processes in the hospital, which
has phases that can be tracked in the real-time experience of the patient and
family. In line 11, the clinician adds to the aura of a routine, predictable process the
further proposition that there is no urgency at the moment, as all curative measures that might cause further suffering have been shown to be unsuccessful. These
gestures appear to take pressure off of the current exchange as a potentially high-
stakes, get-it-right meeting, allowing the clinician to then present Palliative Care
in a rather casual and yet authoritative way below in line 3, citing the volume of
patient visits that the team works with per year. She also describes Palliative Care
not as a group, team, or specialty, but as a "consult service" with diverse function
and wide-ranging clinical presence. The other conversations in this chapter have
not mentioned this latter view about Palliative Care's potential applicability to the
needs of all hospitalized people, a notion that appears aimed toward establishing
credibility.

1 NP: ↑So, we're a ↑consult service, so we do a lot of different things, and in the
2   ↑oncology group. and actually throughout? the hospitals, °we see over
3   1,000 people a year actu[ally.°]
4 Sp: [Yeah.] =↓Yeah
5 NP: °Of any diagnosis° =.hh We ↑help with a bunch of things=↑We help with
6   symptom manage↑ment, (.) so any symptom: we (.) try to help with. .hhh
7 Sp: °Mm-hmm.°
8 NP: We ↑help with ↑goals of care?
9 Sp: °Mm-hmm.°
10 NP: And I think that's <u>actually</u> °everybody.°
11 Sp: Mm-hmm.
12 NP: You know. =finding out (.) what people know about their (.) illness, and how
13   it's affecting them?=What's im<u>portant</u> for them? as far as- well- how they
14   would <u>define</u> a quality of ↓life. .hhhhh
15 Sp: Mm-hmm.

16 NP: And then (.) um (.) what's <u>rea:</u>sonable to <u>try</u> =<°What's <u>rea:</u>sonable
17   to expect.°>
18 Sp: Mm-hmm.
19 NP: And then °just how to help make it so.° (1.2)
20 Sp: Mm-hmm.

In line 11, the clinician expands on her previous gambit of institutional impact and credibility by suggesting that Palliative Care befits the needs of "actually everybody." Her "actually" enhances the sense that the clinician is either thinking through, or *doing* thinking through, the conventional components of Palliative Care together with the family member and coming to new, spontaneous and therefore authentic conclusions based on this interaction itself (on miratives, see DeLancey 2001). This build-up from enumeration to insight can be understood rhetorically and performatively at once – as a strategy of re-presentation and as a moment of identity-formation for the clinician in an as yet relatively young health specialty. She then takes the opportunity in line 13 above to characterize the work of Palliative Care as beneficial for third-person-plural constituency, a "they," which creates some distance from the immediate, intense current situation of suffering that the family is experiencing. This is interesting, because the deictic distance (i.e., the selection of "they" over "you") seems to allow the clinician more freedom to pursue the project of presenting Palliative Care in a way that is not seen as bearing immediately on the perceived needs of the patient, and is therefore able to succeed with a more effective range of portrayal in the interaction.

The suggestion in line 19, that Palliative Care tries to figure out what is reasonable to try and to expect, and to "make it so," is a fascinating formulation, because it plays both on and against the curative, magic-like discourses of hospital medicine, where the institution is expected to cure all woes and ills. The clinician here appears to be trading on that discourse, but reframing it in terms of the rational conduct of Palliative Care in particular situations of suffering and need. She continues:

1 NP: Uh that's a <u>big</u> thing =We do a lot of <u>patient</u> and family sup:port.=We have
2   mas<u>sage</u> <therapy> we have a <u>Reiki</u> therapist.=we- .hh >we have a lot of< (.)
3   ↑nice things.
4 Sp: Yeah.
5 NP: That °you don't always see in° the hospital.
6 Sp: Okay. Good.
7 NP: But (.) we're ↑<u>most</u>ly here: to help you in any way we can.
8 Sp: Mm-hmm. (0.5)

In lines 1–3 above, the clinician expands on the discourse of magically "making it so" and extends it into a "spa" idiom of luxury, pleasure, and therapeutic recovery, a rhetorical move that has not emerged in any of the other conversations we have surveyed in this chapter. Having "nice things" like a Reiki therapist is, of course, one potential way to talk about quality-of-life in a way that people intuitively understand and value.

To summarize, this version of the project "presenting Palliative Care" differs from the others above in that it both majoritizes Palliative Care and scales it to the entire hospital, while 'rarefying' Palliative Care's "nice things" that "you don't often see in the hospital." The nurse practitioner explains that Palliative Care is a "consult service" – rather than, for instance, a group or a "team" – that sees more than 1000 people in the hospital a year. She further asserts that: "We help with goals of care. And I think that's actually everybody." This, combined with naming approximate statistics and the institutional role "consult service" serves to concretize, normalize, and majoritize Palliative Care, rather than minimizing it or allowing it to remain ambiguous in the mind of the patient.

*For further examples of **majoritizing stances on Palliative Care**, see 2.4. For **discussions of urgency**, see 10.11. For **characterizations of Palliative Care as attractive or luxurious**, see 8.4. For strategic **deictic shifts**, see. 2.3.*

2.6 The whole education process

The question that we pursue in this last conversation in Chapter Two is: how do family members or patients understand the immediate relevance of "presenting Palliative Care," and how do they understand the function of that presentation?

The patient in the following conversation self-identifies as a 68-year-old Asian woman and as financially secure, reporting middle-school-level education and Hindu religious affiliation. She has been diagnosed with a stage-four stomach cancer. She believes she is "unlikely" to live for a year, while her clinician-rated survival prognosis is 24 hours to two weeks. In fact, she continued to live for 4 days after this interview, which means that both her own and the clinicians' prognosis estimate were accurate. She strongly ranks her end-of-life goals as "comfort over longevity" and rates her "global" quality-of-life over the previous two days at a two out of ten. The following portion of talk occurred during the first visit of the Palliative Care team, close to the beginning of the conversation. The clinician speaking in the recording is a medical student.

1 MS: I think it might be a good idea to let you rest a little bit.
2 Son: ↑Mom about how much- how much- do you want to (1.5) ↑make a lot of
3   deci↓sions =or do you want to (.) Dad to ((background murmurs))

4 Pt: Wha:t?

5 Son: Do ↑you want to make a lot of de<u>cisions</u>? =or do you want <u>Dad</u> to really

6   (1.2) uh (.) make the decisions.

7 MS: °Make the decisions.°

8 Pt: <u>Dad</u> make °the de↓cisions.°

9 Son: ↑Dad (0.5) talk to- talk to the ↑doctors and then talk °to you.° (1.0)

10 Pt: ((inaudible))

11 Son: ↓Yeah. ↑I don't think she's <u>that</u> interested °in the whole educa↓tion

12   process.°

13 MS: ↑Fair enough.

14 Son: I <u>think</u> I mean- I don't=>You can ask her<Do you want to <u>learn</u> about a:ll

15   this (0.5) ↑hospice and what that ↑is?

16 Pt: Not right-

17 Son: <u>Later</u>?

18 MS: °Yeah.°

19 Pt: I love but I don't think (0.2) I can wake up too lo:ng. I'm uh ( ) like five >or

20   ten minute so can sleep,<

21 MS: You want <u>fi:ve,</u> or ten minutes

22   [so you can sleep?]

23 Son: [She wants a ↓break] I think.

24 MS: Yeah. So I think we should (.)

25   [<u>take</u> a break.]

26 Son: [Let's <u>take</u> a break.]

27 MS: Okay.

28 Pt: I cannot uh- continue talking talking talking ( ).

29 MS: I know (.) sometimes (.) sometimes my voice will: (.) has that

30   <u>soo</u>:thing ef↓fect.

31 Pt: Yeah.

32 MS: Sometimes, not really.

33 Pt: °Yeah? that's right.°

34 MS: ((laughter)) hh

35 Son: °Sometimes too soothingly°. hh ((chuckles))

36 MS: And I'm o↑kay with that <if you're okay with that.>

37 Pt: °Yeah I'm okay too.°

For a number of reasons, the patient's son is trying to close out this conversation before it gets going, convinced that the re-presentation of Palliative Care is as such irrelevant for the patient herself, who – as he seeks to verify in lines 2–6 – has delegated decision-making to her husband, the speaker's father. Here, the patient's son associates Palliative Care with "a lot of decisions" and then recasts it, in lines

11–12, as "the whole education process." He thus anticipates the Palliative Care consultation as the conveyance of an external body of knowledge – rather than, say, as a guide for practical action under current circumstances. This suggests that previous clinicians may have presented Palliative Care in too abstract or educational terms – as interesting and important in its own right, but tangential to the needs of the immediate moment.

Alternately, this exchange shows how, in actual conversations, participants can have differentiated and delegated levels of interest in various aspects of the Palliative Care consultation and will organize the social context of the talk accordingly. Here, the son himself assumes for the group the appropriate quotient of interest in the "whole educational process," delegating to his father "a lot of decisions" and to his mother "resting." This is indeed a complex symbolic triaging procedure in itself, and one that the clinician could potentially have confirmed, in the moment, as reasonable strategies for promoting comfort, alleviation of suffering, and ensuring quality-of-life—the mainstays of Palliative Care as they are often enumerated. Rather, the medical student appears pre-occupied by the son's resistance to the re-presentation genre, and focuses self-deprecatingly on her own persona in the exchange. In line 29–30, she attempts a repair to her own threatened positive face, upon the patient's insistence that she cannot "continue talking talking talking." The medical student's repair ensues by shifting persona away from her position as representative of Palliative Care, and toward her own speaking voice, which she frames positively as "soothing" (line 30). The patient's son supports this repair in line 35, assisting the medical student in conferring positive face upon herself for the purpose of alleviating the threat to positive face in line 11 and 28.

The broader question is, perhaps, to what extent does a clinician's positive face, whether as a representative of Palliative Care or of the medical establishment of the hospital, pertain in this equation of relieving suffering and improving quality in an end-of-life context. As we noted in the patient profile, this woman survived for four days after this consultation, which was within both clinical and family prognosis expectations. How, then, can the presentation of Palliative Care offerings be modulated to mitigate the objective social need for face recognition that clinicians (whether medical students or attending physicians) implicitly introduce into a conversation like this? Are there ways to preempt or obviate some of the politeness rituals that the patient's son undertakes here – perhaps by foregoing any form of frontal presentation whatsoever?

*For further examples of **delegating symbolic responsibilities**, see 7.4, 8.2, 8.3. For **characterizations of Palliative Care as "educational"**, see 3.5. For **exhaustion with talking in general**, see 3.1, 3.4. For **clinician self-deprecation**, see 9.5.*

2.7 Insights and implications from Chapter 2

From these conversations, it becomes clear that no script, monologue, or dialogical sequencing can claim to encapsulate an ideal model of this speech genre of introducing Palliative Care. Rather, the granular contingency of each individual patient and context will prevail in the meaning-making process of interaction. Still, we see some vectors of talk that are salient: sometimes patients and families have good reason to stall or derail the re-presentation project; sometimes clinicians find ways to render Palliative Care as a discipline attractive without being overbearing. Often, successful presentations of Palliative Care are those that appear less patient-centered on their surface (i.e. less explicitly oriented toward the "you" of interaction) and more reliant on a distanced, abstracted "they" that refers to seriously-ill people who have found Palliative Care services helpful in past instances. Furthermore, patients' bids for the recognition of their own epistemic status as "familiar", as "a silent partner," or as a negotiator appear to be important to the successful co-creation of the presentation. While this current chapter focused primarily on clinician-centered characterizations, the next chapter shifts the focus onto how patients query these clinical characterizations for various purposes.

3 Querying Palliative Care

If there are various and often conflicting interactional manifestations of the "representing Palliative Care" project in consultations, there is an equally vibrant range of ways in which patients and family members see fit to poke around in these presentations as they are conveyed. All branches of health care are subject to curiosity, skepticism, and inquiry on the part of patients and families, who attempt in various ways to understand where one discipline ends and where another begins, as well as the underlying motivations and beliefs clinicians bring about the world, about health, about them as human beings. There are very practical questions, too, arising from the idiom of specialization in medicine. Is Palliative Care a specialty in the way that oncology is a specialty? Or, if a cancer is metastasized throughout the body, it will be rational for patients to seek clarification about whether that cancer is being treated primarily under the clinical aegis of oncologists or, say, of pulmonologists.

In the United States, the case is somewhat more complex because the Palliative Care discipline, its board-certified status, and its structural position within hospitals are still quite new. Many if not most of the patients presented in this book began to seek health care for serious illness *before* most hospitals had a dedicated Palliative Care service. Thus, their questions, whether asked or unasked, will include not only traditional uncertainties about turf and territory amongst medical disciplines, but about the discipline's fundamental purpose and rationale – questions that most cardiologists, for instance, are only seldom asked to field in comprehensive ways.

In this chapter we present and analyze conversations in which patients or families query Palliative Care for one reason or another. Sometimes patients' conversational projects to query Palliative Care are informational and straightforward, while other times the project is social and discriminating, designed to ritually incorporate as-yet-unknown social relations into a vernacular landscape. We also include in this chapter instances in which patients and families abstain from querying Palliative Care when such a query seems most appropriate, and we attempt to indicate what the consequences of that interactional abstention can be.

3.1 How many people are in Palliative Care?

The questions that motivate us to present the first conversation in this chapter on querying Palliative Care are as follows:
1) How do patients and families, as yet unfamiliar with Palliative Care as a branch of medicine, test and probe it in various ways that are not directly informational?

https://doi.org/10.1515/9781501504570-003

2) Are such testing-and-probing projects on the part of patients ritualistic and phatic (i.e., designed for establishing contact or "small talk") or do they appear to have broader ideological implications?

The patient in the following conversation self-identifies as an 85-year-old white man and as financially secure, reporting graduate-level education and Christian religious affiliation. He has been diagnosed with a stage-four prostate cancer. He believes he is "very likely" to live for a year, while his clinician-rated survival prognosis at the time of the following consultation is six months. In fact, he lived 78 days beyond this consultation, i.e., shorter than both the clinical expectation and his own. The patient strongly ranks his end-of-life goals as "comfort over longevity," and he rates his "global" quality-of-life over the previous two days at a six out of ten. The following portion of talk occurred during the first visit of the Palliative Care team. The clinicians speaking in the conversation are a Palliative Care physician and a PC nurse practitioner.

1	Pt:	How many <u>pe</u>ople are in ((chair scraping the floor)) Palliadiv-↑PalliaTive
2		↑Care? (0.5)
3	NP:	Like our ↑whole depart↑<u>ment</u>?
4	Pt:	Yeah.
5	NP:	A ↑lot of us:.
6	Pt:	I know. (0.5) >We almost came down there about two years ago.< (0.5)
7	MD:	Dozen or so? ((chairs moving))
8	NP:	More than <u>that</u>.=I think we have ten or so at<u>ten</u>ding:s plus three <u>fellows</u>:
9		>[↑I don't know 16 17?]<
10	MD:	[When you add everyone ( )]
11	Pt:	You guys do a <u>hell</u> of a lot of maintenance too because our our ↑son had
12		ah ↑throat cancer (0.8)
13	MD:	Ah::.

The arranging and scraping of chairs and movement in the space mirrors the bearing of the patient's orienting question, in which he engages in a kind of polite 'forces assessment inventory' about Palliative Care, i.e., "how *many* people are you". This emphasis on quantity and 'manpower' will become salient again later in the interaction, when the patient talks about his own strength in a physical altercation. The patient's self-correction in line 1, repronouncing "palliaTive" the second time with a plosive t, does not indicate unfamiliarity with the specialty, but rather indexes the patient's slightly ironic, quizzically honorific stance through the hyper-correct enunciation of the word. In line 1, the "how many people" question initiates complex dynamics of pre-alignment and pre-affiliation (Lindström 2009), and the two clinicians' responses are variously dysfluent in their accommodation of it (Barton 2006; Dwamena et al. 2012; Emanuel and Emanuel 1992; Hesson et al. 2012; Johnson et al. 2000). While they are perhaps intuitively well-inclined to answer the preferred question *What is Palliative Care?* or *What does Palliative Care offer?*, they do not spontaneously regard this question of quantity in staffing and personnel as relevant. The implicature of the nurse practitioner's first emphatic response in line 5, which flouts the Gricean maxim of Quantity, appears to be that the patient does not need to know such back-of-the-house detail, though she does introduce previously in line 3 the institutional idiom of "department" in pursuit of clarification. This delay-and-regroup sequence in lines 3–5 ends when the patient responds "I know" and continues on to account for his own experiences with Palliative Care, while seeking treatment for his own son's illness in the recent past. The meaning of the patient's word "maintenance" in line 11, where the patient gives positive face to the group through the emphatic "hell of a lot of *maintenance*", is not entirely clear. What does the patient mean by maintenance, and what is maintenance's relationship to other types of hospital practice – like treatment, curing disease, consulting, etc.? The patient elaborates on his prior experiences with his son's illness:

1 Pt: And ↑he was <u>almost</u> sent ↑down there two years a↓go.
2 MD: ↓Mm hmm. (0.5)
3 Pt: And we said naa: >°let's keep him up here and they did°.<
4 Sp: So ↑this looks like it might ↑take a while, ((laughter))
5 MD: Well?
6 Pt: No not really,
7 MD: <u>We're</u> gonna <u>we're</u> gonna-
8 Pt: What am I gonna ↑do? (0.2) ((laughter))
9 NP: Do you ↑have other plans?
10 NP2: Do you have a <u>tee</u>-↑time at a-
11 Pt: Let me ↑check my sche↓dule.
12 NP2: That's right? (0.8) Well we we no we're <u>here</u> for <u>you</u> (0.2) Um:: and of
13   course our area of exper<u>tise</u> is in Palliative ↓Care so we're we're to help
14   with <u>symptom</u> ma↑<u>nagement</u> [...]

The patient's incipient telling in lines 1 and 3 is interesting for its deictic projections; "here" is ambiguous because it indexes both the non-Palliative Care floor where the patient's son had been treated two years prior, but also the "here" of the non-Palliative Care setting where the current patient is now being seen, and where he is considering whether or not to avail himself of the Palliative Care team's services. The patient's turn in line 3 appears to indicate the project behind his telling, i.e., that Palliative Care was unnecessary in the treatment of his son's cancer and that insights won from such judgment of necessity will likely inform his current decision-making. But any telling about the further development of their son's treatment is aborted, as the patient's spouse interrupts his telling abruptly with a proposal of a new topic, which is a metadiscursive query about the Palliative Care consultation, namely whether it will *take a while* (in line 4). This off-record face threat toward the clinical team's bearing is immediately redressed by the patient himself, either with the implicature that he feels equipped to expedite the conversation, that in his experience Palliative Care consultations are unburdensome, or that he wishes to project general magnanimity.

In fact, seeing the physician struggle to regain footing, the patient mitigates the face threat even further in line 8 with the comic crystallization of affairs "What [else] am I gonna do?", recycling the physician's forecasting token "gonna" from the previous turn. The patient's overall project in this section of talk, from his original query about "how many people" to his mitigation of his spouse's face-threat, appears to be that of someone giving a potential adversary a fair shake. The techniques involved include asking open-ended questions that allow the interlocutors to present themselves to their satisfaction before, perhaps, dismissing them – as the patient intimates in the telling of his son's story in line 3. The sequence in which various participants (the physician, nurse practitioner, and patient) explore the metaphor of scheduling – at the expense of his spouse's intervention about the consultation potentially *taking a while* – opens up a phenomenon frequently on view in these interactions generally. Patients and clinicians frequently and playfully evoke resources of leisure, business, golf, and the patient's busy schedule despite the fact that, in this patient's case as in others, he will spend the remaining weeks of his life negotiating his health care needs, rather than having a tee-time. The extent to which these metaphorical resources of the imagination (about freedom, leisure, sports, the outdoors, roaming, etc.) are a crucial idiom for the Palliative Care consultation and its holistic, normalizing quality-of-life goals will continue to become evident in conversations that follow.

*For further examples of **the time burden of consultations**, see 2.6, 3.4. For **patients' attempts to vet Palliative Care personnel**, see 2.1, 5.4. For idioms of **leisure and the outdoors**, see 4.1, 5.4. For patients' **reflection on others' prior experiences with palliative modalities**, see 3.2, 3.5, 4.2, 5.5.*

3.2 I can't speak to your father's case for sure

In contrast to the previous conversation, this exchange below between a patient and Palliative Care clinician appears to proceed neither along ritual and phatic terrain, nor does it respond to a patient's need for information, but rather addresses a profound existential and moral question the patient has long ruminated upon. As with conversation 3.1, this patient has had a previous experience with palliative modalities of care, and is – unlike the case in 3.1 – haunted by its implications and outcome. The patient, who is struggling with persistent shortness of breath due to her lung cancer, is considering accepting palliative treatment that would ease her symptoms but perhaps also decrease her physiological persistence. The physicians here are explaining how pain-relief/symptom-management medications work, and this explanation prompts the patient to reflect on a previous experience of symptom management she experienced while caring for her dying father, at a time when the discipline of Palliative Medicine did not yet exist in the United States. She thus views her own decision-making horizon about any incipient Palliative Care treatments through the lens of those her father experienced a generation previously, seeking moral clarity from the Palliative Care physicians about whether she had, in pursuing comfort measures for her father, "killed" him.

The questions that motivate our reflections here are thus as follows:

1) What kinds of moral, existential, and family-historical questions do patients pose to Palliative Care specialists, and what experiences prompt them to do so?
2) How do Palliative Care practitioners formulate answers to such questions that, even when they are topically not "about" the patient's disease, can nonetheless play an important role in improving that patient's current quality-of-life, wholeness, and comfort?
3) How do Palliative Care clinicians address historical discourses like "mercy killing," when these themes and idioms are raised by patients?

The patient in this conversation self-identifies as a 66-year-old white woman and as financially secure, reporting Associate's-level education and Christian religious affiliation. She has been diagnosed with a stage-four lung cancer. She believes she is "very likely" to live for a year, while her clinician-rated survival prognosis at the time of the following consultation is two weeks to three months. In fact, she lived 11 days beyond this consultation, i.e., shorter than clinically expected and much shorter than she herself expected at the time. The patient is unsure whether comfort or longevity is more important to her at the moment, and she rates her "global" quality-of-life over the previous two days at a three out of ten. The following portion of talk occurred during the first visit of the Palliative Care team. The clinicians speaking are a Palliative Care attending physician and a Palliative Care physician fellow.

The patient is asking the fellow and physician here to speculate on how her father's process of dying was clinically overseen, and whether a "third shot" of morphine administered to him constituted what she understands as a "mercy killing." Seeing a question that requires a particular delicacy in response, the physician steps in in line 6–9 below and "steals the thunder" from the PC fellow (i.e. an advanced trainee) who is not entirely prepared to respond to the patient's elliptical formulation of the event of her father's passing. This is one instance, common in Palliative Care interactional contexts, where a patient's shortness of breath conflicts with her desire to express herself in as comprehensive and articulate a way as possible about the topic she initiates. This common feature exacerbates potential asymmetries in air-time between clinicians and patients, and leads less experienced clinicians to precipitously interrupt out of a desire to help the patient get her thoughts out. We note that such an exacerbation does not appear to take place here, as the physician's longer explanation is punctuated by very frequent pauses and micro-pauses that invite and acknowledge nodding or other forms of non-verbal confirmation from the patient, indicating she is following the physician's line of thought quite closely.

```
1  Pt:   Would they would they have ↑done that with him? ↑asked him? (0.5)
2         ((beeping)) if he wanted help? (1.2)
3  Fel:  Would they have done which part of it. (0.5)
4  Pt:   The- you >know when they did the third shot?< (0.7)
5  MD:   It's a good question=Let me let me (0.2) try to answer that. =It's it's a
6         tough one. (1.0) The: (.) what what you're just saying = And ((referring
7         to the fellow)) I'm stealing your thunder again.=and you can step on my
8         toes in a mo↓ment.
9  Fel:  No,
10 MD:   Uh- (0.8) it's all about the intention. (0.8) And the intention- and I ↑can't
11        speak to your father's case for sure (0.5) but I will tell you our practice:
12        (0.2) and we have a lot of (.) practice with ↓this (.) ↓here ((beeping))
13        (0.5) is to treat (0.5) ↑your: (0.6) or anyone else's symptoms- treat your
14        shortness of breath to the extent you wish:. (1.0) As much (.) as you need
15        to feel >as comfortable as you need.< (0.5) There are situations in which
16        (0.2) a bit more medication (0.2) ↑will ((beeping)) be e↑nough (0.5) to
17        make someone s:o comfortable so relaxed that they actually stop breathing.
18        (1.0) They ↑could ↓die. (0.2) It's ↑not the intention.=That's ↑not the goal:.
19        (0.2) We ↑will not intend to do ↓that. (0.5) We will give as much medication
20        ↑like the ↑morphine, (0.8) as you wish ((beeping)) for your com↓fort. (0.8)
21        And with advanced lung di↓sease (0.2) it can re↑quire (0.2) a fair amount
22        of this medicine (0.2) and it could make you very peacefully relaxed. (0.5)
```

23   It is ↑possible (0.8) that it would make you so re↓laxed (0.8) that your
24   breathing would slow e↓nough (0.5) that you would ↑die: soo↓ner. (0.2)
25   It's possible. (0.2) It's not how we're intending to use it. (0.2) And as long
26   as ↑you know this (0.5) you can request essentially as much medication as
27   you need for your comfort, (0.8) Does ↑that make sense?
28 Pt: °Yes.°

The experienced Palliative Care attending physician, seeing that his fellow/trainee
is struggling to accommodate the informational, moral, existential, and clinical
import of the patient's question in line 1 about her father's end-of-life experience,
steps in resolutely but politely. The long explanation from lines 10–27 is made up of
short paratactical sentences with frequent pauses to invite interruptions. The physician uses a diversity of deictic frames ("you", "they", "someone") to dramatize
what happens when morphine is used to alleviate symptoms, such as the shortness
of breath the patient is having (see also Anderson and Keenan 1985; Aikhenvald
2004; Fillmore 1997; Fretheim et al. 2011). In line 11, the physician states that he
cannot speak to the patient's father's experience, but he then nonetheless narrates
in good detail the sequences and contingencies that most often take place in a scenario much like her father's. He adroitly blends the sequence and decision-making
rhythm of her father's case with the potential course of her own Palliative Care
treatment, not focusing overlong on comparing or distinguishing the two cases.

Importantly, too, the physician continues to describe these sequences in a
way that is directly applicable to the patient's current clinical circumstances.
Thus far in this chapter, the two ways in which patients query "Palliative Care"
are based in patients' own past experiences of others' serious illnesses, and on
their previous interactions with clinical strategies that would today be referred to
as "palliative," but were perhaps not in previous generations. Patients bring their
own vernacular knowledge and experiences of these settings with them, and the
further question arises:

4) How can these past experiences be best engaged as a resource for current
   clinical, social, spiritual, and interactional needs?

The attending Palliative Care physician continues his account:

1 MD: Okay (.) so we can't speak to exactly what happened with your fa↓ther. (0.5)
2   I have ↑not witnessed (0.2) us in this practice or others who do this work
3   (0.8) giving more and more and more medicine (0.2) hoping that last one
4   will ↓end it. (0.5) That's ↑not the way this is inten↓ded.
5 Pt: 'Cause ↑it's just something (1.0) that's ↑always ↑bothered ↓me about
6   my dad.

7 MD: I can see it.

8 Pt: Did- did I <u>kill</u> him? (0.2)

9 MD: ↓Yeah. (1.2) °I can ↓see.° (0.5) I can <u>see</u> it. (0.5) ↑My sus<u>picion</u> ↑is (0.2)

10   you saw he was un<u>com</u>fortable, (0.8) my suspicion is you wanted him to be

11   <u>rest</u>ful: (0.5) and not uncomfor<u>table</u> (0.8) and then he died. (1.2) Was that

12   be<u>cause</u> of the medicine?=Was it as a result of his getting more comfortable?

13   (0.2) I ↑can't know for sure,

After the physician's account, the patient brings the focus back to her experience with her father as "something that's always bothered me." Importantly, the physician acknowledges this concern with the repeated phrase "I can see it," but does not take over from the patient the moral responsibility to decide whether she killed him or not. He does not say, for instance, "My suspicion is that you did not kill him." Rather, he describes the process, the intention, and the decision-making protocols that likely lead to his death, and leaves this portrayal for the patient to evaluate on her own terms.

The physician's selection of "not uncomfortable" in line 11 above is interesting, because it replaces the more common discursive trope "not in pain" that often peppers tellings of physician- or family-assisted suicide. The idea, however, that death can be a result of one's "getting more comfortable" is a unique and powerful formulation here in line 12 which, given that this patient herself died 11 days after this conversation, itself has important palliative benefits for her in this setting.

For further examples of **reflection on others' prior experiences with palliative modalities,** *see 3.1, 3.5, 4.2, 5.5. For* **patients' moral concern about hastening death,** *see 6.2, 4.4, 4.3, 6.2, 6.4. For* **characterizations of the dying process,** *see 10.1, 4.3, 8.4. 3.6.*

3.3 We're pretty familiar with it

In this third conversation, clinicians again learn in the course of the consultation that patients and family members already have some experience with Palliative Care as a specialty or as an approach. Here, however, this fact emerges not in the form of a query or a telling, but appears to be withheld throughout the initial portion of the interaction. The questions that motivate our analysis here are:

1) How and when do patients and family members forgo disclosure of their previous experiences with Palliative Care?

2) What interactional features prompt them to do so?

The patient in the following conversation self-identifies as a 66-year-old white woman and as financially insecure, reporting Bachelor's-level education and no religious affiliation. She has been diagnosed with a cancer of the peripheral nervous system and spinal cord, which is advanced. She has "no idea" whether she will live for a year, while her clinician-rated survival prognosis at the time of the consultation is three to six months. In fact, she lived more than six months, i.e., longer than the follow-up window of this study and longer than clinicians expected. The patient strongly ranks her end-of-life goals as "comfort over longevity," and she rates her "global" quality-of-life over the previous two days at a six out of ten. The following portion of talk occurred during the first visit of the Palliative Care team. The clinicians speaking are a Palliative Care physician fellow and a Palliative Care nurse practitioner. The patient in this exchange is using a speech-generating device to communicate, and her spouse often interprets for her. In the transcript below, quotation marks surround those utterances that participants directly quote and repeat on the patient's behalf as they interpret the device-generated speech that, though inaudible on the recording, could be heard in the interactional space.

1 Fel: And so what I'm sort of alluding to↑ (0.5) we have um a way of delivering
2   care: for people (0.2) at home or in a place that's ↑not the hospi↑tal (0.5)
3   that would be focused on (0.5) keeping: (0.2) someone as comfor↓table as
4   possible. ((inaudible, 2.00)) "What is ↑this place?" (2.2) "Hospice?" (0.5)
5   Hospice is what I'm referring to yeah. (1.8)
6 Sp: °"We're pretty familiar with it,"°
7 Fel: Are you familiar with ↑that? (3.0)
8 NP: "We have one up there," (1.8)
9 Sp: °She volunteers.°
10 Sp: [°"I'm a hospice Chaplain."°]
11 Fel: [You're the ↑hospice Chap↑lain?]
12 Sp: [Yeah,] she was.
13 Pt: [°Yeah. °]
14 Fel: No way, ((laughter))
15 NP: You didn't ↑tell me that ((laughter)) (0.5)
16 Fel: After right after meeting you, >do you know, it's like< we really have a
17   lot in common. ((laughter)) Your actual occupation, ((laughter)) That's
18   hilarious, ((laughter)) (0.2) and awesome. (.) Amazing. >So it is exactly
19   what I'm referring to?< (.) Uh and I don't know if that is what makes
20   sense at this moment or >if would make sense in the fu↓ture but I
21   think you definitely should (.) ↑think about ↓that as something in

22   our tool↓kit as something ↓that is a way (.) ↓uh (.) that (0.5) we can
23   res<u>pond</u> to e<u>mergen</u>↑cies: (.) that wouldn't be going to the Emergency
24   ↓Room. (3.5)
25 Pt: °Mm-hmm.°

Two clinician-initiated sections of this exchange in lines 1–6 and 19–25 belong to the "re-presenting Palliative Care" genre addressed in Chapter 2. There is on the clinician's part a predominance of hedging, indirection, and stylized presentational lexicon, which includes such common phrases of the genre as "in our toolkit," "what makes sense," etc. At the beginning of this presentational volley, the physician fellow talks of hospice as "what I'm sort of alluding to", which is a formulation involving double indirection – i.e., "sort of" and "alluding to", giving the impression that hospice itself must necessarily be by nature a difficult topic to address directly, requiring significant buffering and handling in the course of its presentation. Of course, since the patient is using a speech-generating device, her capacity to engage in indirection, hedging, contextualization cues, and epistemic markers in customary ways is significantly curtailed, and this asymmetry of discourse-marking resources between clinician and patient is a rather regular phenomenon within Palliative Care interactions (Ariss 2009; Maynard 1991; Delancey 2001; Drew 1991; Eagan and Weatherson 2011; Enfield 2011; Foucault 1980; ten Have 1991; Heritage 2012; see also Kamio 1997; Lindström and Weatherall 2015; Pilnick and Dingwall 2011). Put another way, clinicians are able to euphemize using various genres and styles with more intricacy and flexibility than many patients are able or willing to do – precisely because they are constrained by physiological symptoms or side-effects of treatment.

What seems remarkable in this exchange is that, though the patient (using a speech-generating device) interrupts the clinician's presentational roll-out of the idea of hospice, announcing that she herself is a hospice chaplain (only after the pre-announcement "we're pretty familiar with it" (in line 6), the clinician does not alter course accordingly. There is an extended sequence of repair from line 11 to 17, in which the fellow praises the patient and offers a great-minds-think-alike gesture, but then the clinician returns to the presentation genre script, even though there is no remaining interactional or substantive reason to do so. This is, we believe, an instance in which some of the stylistic and genre conventions of "presenting Palliative Care" may tend to impede patients' ability to effectively share their own level of understanding and involvement. Certainly, the speech-generating technology may have played a role in discouraging the clinician from inviting the patient to narrate from her experiences and insights as a hospice chaplain, but the clinical benefit of doing so would seem to have far outweighed the interactional costs. That is, learning from the patient what knowledge and wisdom she has gained from her work as a hospice professional would increase the overall interactional and thematic resources available to the participants in this consultation, and to any ensuing palliative treatment plan.

For further examples of **patients declining to disclose some aspect of their identities**, see 2.3, 9.3, 6.3. For the **predominance of hedging and indirection**, see 3.3, 6.1, 6.2, 7.3. For **patients whose physiological constraints lead them to formulate ideas frankly**, see 4.5, 6.1.

3.4 How long do I have to go through this

The following conversation is an instance in which the patient is refusing uptake of Palliative Care as an option for his treatment, while the clinical team remains predisposed to see the patient's contributions as potential openings for a prognosis and goals-of-care conversation. The patient here self-identifies as a 69-year-old white man and as financially secure, reporting high-school-level education and Christian religious affiliation. He has been diagnosed with a stage-four colon cancer. He is unsure of his prognosis, while his clinician-rated survival prognosis at the time of the following consultation is three to six months. There is no record of his length of survival past this consultation. The patient strongly ranks his end-of-life goals as "longevity over comfort," and he rates his "global" quality-of-life over the previous two days at eight out of ten. The following portion of talk occurred during the first visit of the Palliative Care team. The clinicians speaking are a Palliative Care attending physician and a Palliative Care physician fellow. The topic under consideration at this point in the conversation is quality-of-life, pain, and acceptable levels of discomfort, given the patient's stage-four colon cancer and its symptoms. The clinicians are asking him to identify a level of pain that he can live with and still experience quality-of-life, with 10 as the highest level of pain possible.

1 MD: >What would be your goal.< (1.5)
2 Pt: Number?
3 MD: ↑Yeah. (0.5)
4 Pt: Nine, (0.5)
5 MD: What would be a ↑good number for you? =What would be a (.) an
6   acceptable (0.2) number that you could live at? (0.2)
7 Pt: ↓Ni:ne. (0.8)
8 MD: So you can
9   [live with it the way it is   ] now?
10 MD: [Nine. >So you can live with a nine?<]
11 Pt: ↓Yeah.

12 MD: All right. (1.0)
13 Fel: You're a tough guy. (2.0)
14 MD: °That's true.° ((chuckles)) (0.2) hhhh Is that true?
15 Pt: Yeah, I guess so.
16 MD: Yeah. (0.5) >Are you ↑up walking a↑round a little bit?<
17 Pt: A lit↓tle.
18 MD: A little bit. (0.2) °Okay°. (2.0) All right. (0.8)
19   Questions you got at all for ↑us. (1.0)
20 Pt: How long (1.2) do I go through (.) th- this? (0.5)
21 MD: You ↓mean (0.8) you're asking about how <u>long</u> do you <u>have</u> to ↑live.
22 Pt: No, how long do I have to (0.5) go <u>through</u> this <u>ques</u>tioning?
23 Fel: ↑Oh.
24 MD: Questioning can be done right now if you're ↓done.((laughter))
25 Fel: We're done if you:'re done. (0.2)
26 Pt: I'm <u>done</u>.

Despite his "tough" insistence that he can happily handle nine-out-of-ten pain, it appears to the clinicians in lines 21–23 that the patient is, finally, showing some modest interest in the ideas about Palliative Care presented to him in the course of the referral consultation. The clinicians are inclined to view the patient's contributions from within their thematic frame, rather than from the emphatic and strategic stance the patient has taken in lines 7–11, i.e., showing as little interest as possible in the holistic and reflective components of a Palliative Care conversation.

The clinicians initiate in line 20 a pre-closing using a truncated style befitting an aborted project (see Schegloff and Sacks 1973 on closings). The ambiguity of the "this' prompts the clinicians to view the tolerated ordeal the patient is alluding to as his cancer, whereas the patient is intending to query the "questioning" itself. Of course, this particular word "questioning" associates with genres like "inquisition" and "interrogation" much more easily than it does with, say, a medical consultation. Nonetheless, the Palliative Care physician returns the "questioning" token in line 25, granting the patient's associative premise that "this" has been an ordeal of some sort. We do note that this patient is one of the very few among our study who strongly rates "longevity" over "comfort" as the prevailing goal of the treatment of his advanced colon cancer and that he indeed may have lived significantly longer than the clinical prognosis of three to six months.

*For further examples of **clinicians ascribing toughness or strength to patients**, see 4.1, 9.3, 9.1, 5.5. For examples of consultations as a **burden or ordeal**, see 2.6, 3.1.*

3.5 Okay I copyrighted it so you gotta pay me

"Querying Palliative Care" is a project that is not always a patient-/family-initiated query, to which a member of the clinical team responds. Sometimes, as in the following conversation, a query emerges in conversation and is addressed by a family member or the patient herself. For instance, in conversation 3.1, it was the patient who responded to his spouse's concern as to whether the consultation would take a long time, by saying "No not really." The following conversation is an extended instance in which a family member "jumps in" to explain some aspect of the palliative approach, here the philosophy of hospice care. For us, the questions then are:

1) What function and value do family-initiated tellings about Palliative Care (its functions, philosophy, benefits, etc.) offer that clinician-initiated presentations may not?
2) Is this difference primarily dependent on the trust patients show in their own family members' contributions over those of strangers or institutional representatives?
3) Are there ways of speaking and interactional resources that family members take up, which are simply unavailable to clinicians?
4) Can clinical consultations somehow explicitly or formally foster opportunities for such intragroup tellings?

The patient in the following conversation self-identifies as an 80-year-old white man and as financially secure, reporting graduate-level education and no religious affiliation. He has been diagnosed with a stage-four cancer, which has not been biopsied. He believes he is "very unlikely" to live for a year, while his clinician-rated survival prognosis is two weeks to three months. In fact, he continued to live for 34 days after this interview, which means that both his and the clinicians' prognosis estimates were accurate. He ranks his end-of-life goals as "comfort over longevity" and he rates his "global" quality-of-life over the previous two days – physical, emotional, social, spiritual, and financial – at a zero out of ten. The following portion of talk occurred during the first visit of the Palliative Care team, close to the beginning of the conversation. The clinician speaking is a Palliative Care physician.

1 MD: So right now we're kind of talking (.) ↑plan A: (0.5) this is what it would
2   look like.=But if ↑that doesn't work (0.2) then we're going to plan B: or
3   (0.8) plan ↑A (0.8) number two or whatever the case may be.
4 Dt: °Mm-hmm.°
5 Sp: °Mm-hmm.°

6 MD: I mean (0.5) >when people are as sick as you are,< (0.8) m- you always
7   have (0.8) to have be ready to change-
8 Sp: °Mm-hmm.°
9 SiL: I <u>think</u> you're gonna find (0.2) I mean we've all been commen↓ting what
10   good care he's been getting <u>here</u> the last 24 ↓hours. (1.2)
11 Sp: °Mm-hmm.°
12 SiL: ↑My sense <u>is</u>: (2.2) no offense to people ↓here.=↑hospice is going to put
13   °them all to shame° (0.8) Okay?
14 Pt: [Hos- say that again,   ]
15 SiL: [I think you're gonna] (0.2) ↑hospice (.) ↑<u>ho</u>spice is gonna put this
16   care to ↓shame. (0.5)
17 MD: Okay.
18 SiL: ↑Okay? (0.2) And it's (0.8) think of it like of as an ↑hospice is an
19   a↑moebous <u>blob</u>.
20 Sp: °Mm-hmm.°
21 SiL: Your <u>needs</u> ↑change? ↑↑blooop? so does ↓hospice.
22 Dt: I like that you ↑got it.
23 MD: Okay.
24 SiL: Okay I <u>copyrighted</u> it >so you gotta pay me every time you< ((laughter))
25   You know I <u>think</u>? (0.8)
26 Dt: <u>He's</u> an expert now >because of his <u>dad</u>.< ((laughter))
27 SiL: Well '>cos he sits there and ↑talks about it all the time.<
28 Dt: Right. =Yeah.
29 SiL: And I <u>see</u> what ↑he has to do and what-
30 Sp: Mm-hmm,
31 SiL: You know? =it's- it's gonna <u>change</u> with <u>you</u>?
32 Dt: You get <u>cre</u>ative.
33 SiL: And it may be the <u>absolute</u> ↑wrong option?
34 Pt: Yeah.
35 SiL: And then we change the ↓option.
36 Pt: Yeah. (0.8)

At the outset of this portion of the consultation, the physician is completing his own thorough presentation of the various care scenarios available to a seriously-ill patient. In line 9, the patient's son-in-law seeks to extend, rather than contradict the physician's account, ascribing to hospice care an extraordinary adaptability. Where the physician in lines 6–7 had formulated the need for flexibility and readiness for change as a characteristic required of the patient (here the explicit "you", though "you" might well extend to the family generally), the son-in-law reformulates the physician's account by presenting his own metaphor of the amoeba of hospice as a service that *itself* offers the characteristic of flexibility, thus taking this symbolic burden off the patient. Such tag-team alignments between clinicians and family members in the endeavor to illustrate potential treatment scenarios can engender new levels of solidarity, and indeed the son-in-law's stroke-of-genius contribution of the amoeba metaphor enables him to claim a kind of lay-expert position that he jokes about in line 24, while his wife attributes it to her father-in-law's experience and wisdom. This is interesting, because it evokes a chiastic honorific kinship relation in which the daughter gives face to *her* (absent) father-in-law, while the son-in-law offers his lay expertise to *his* father-in-law. Meanwhile, the physician is content to attend this telling as an appreciative bystander, without seeking to direct or correct any of the family's intragroup illustrations as they query Palliative Care together.

For further examples of **patients and families creating their own character-izations of Palliative Care**, see *8.1, 5.3, 2.3, 10.7, 5.4*.

3.6 Do they get to drink and eat?

We close this chapter with a representative conversation that foregrounds what is, in our experience, one of the most typically substantive ways in which patients and family members query Palliative Care and hospice philosophy in our study. Beyond testing-and-prodding questions geared toward social and other status-acknowledgement goals, there are a few questions that are consistently important for families, enough so that they will pose them even in interactionally inopportune moments (Azoulay et al. 2003; Curtis et al. 2002; Curtis et al. 2001; Heyland et al. 2003; Kirchhoff et al. 2002; see also Stivers 2007). For us, then, the current conversation answers the question:

1) What items tend to be foremost in family members' minds about the nuts-and-bolts of Palliative Care, but are often not quite made clear to them in "re-presenting Palliative Care" volleys?

The patient in the following conversation self-identifies as an 86-year-old white woman and as financially secure, reporting high-school-level education and no religious affiliation. She has been diagnosed with a stage-four ovarian cancer. She has "no idea" about her own prognosis, while her clinician-rated survival prognosis at the time of the following consultation is two weeks to three months. In fact, she lived 38 days beyond this consultation, i.e., within clinical expectations. The patient is unsure whether her end-of-life goal is "comfort" or "longevity," and she rates her "global" quality-of-life over the previous two days at a five out of ten. The following portion of talk occurred during the second visit of the Palliative Care team. The clinician speaking is a Palliative Care physician.

1 MD: So (.) _____ it's it's (.) ↑more important to think (.) first of hospice as
2   (0.2) hospice is an i↑dea. =It's a way to <u>care</u> for a patient as opposed to
3   an <u>ac</u>tual ↓place. (0.5)
4 Pt: Right.
5 MD: The place comes la↓ter.
6 Pt: Right.
7 MD: ↑First think of ↓it as (.) here's how we're going to approach this ill↓ness.
8   (0.5) And (.) the <u>main:</u> idea of it is (0.2) that instead of saying we're going
9   to ↑<u>take</u> what's ↑bother- what's making you <u>sick</u> and try to ↑<u>cure:</u> it? (1.0)
10   the idea is (.) let's try to make what's making you <u>feel</u> so bad (.) feel
11   better.=Let's make the symptoms feel <u>bet</u>ter.
12 Pt: Oh ↑I agree with that,
13 MD: And and that often means that we don't do things that (0.6) pro<u>long</u> your
14   life artificially,
15 Pt: Right,
16 MD: We don't do things like (0.5) >put people on <u>breath</u>ing ma↑chines.<
17 Pt: °Right. °
18 MD: We don't give them medications to keep their <u>blood</u> pressure ↑up.=We
19   don't give them dialy↓sis. =>things like that.<
20 Pt: Right.
21 MD: We ↑give them things (0.3) for ↑what they're feeling. =Am I feeling pain.
22   (0.2) =We treat the pain.
23 Pt: Right.
24 MD: They're having nausea we treat the nau↓sea.
25 Pt: Right.
26 MD: Anxiety and >↑so on and ↑so on.< (0.5) But it is oriented <u>to</u>wards dealing
27   with those (.) <u>symp</u>toms (0.2) and trying to make a patient ↑<u>comfort</u>able as
28   opposed to saying ↑Let's (.) <u>cure:</u> (.) what's (.) making you sick.
29 Pt: °Right. °
30 MD: Even at the expense of making you feel ↓worse.

This conversation exhibits a version of the re-presenting Palliative Care genre that is predominantly negative, in the sense of defining the treatment based on what it does *not* do. The patient appears to follow this account quite closely, offering acknowledgement tokens frequently throughout. The first intervention comes from a family member at this point:

1 FM: Do they get to ↑drink (.) and eat:?
2 MD: ↑Absolutely. (0.3) A ↑big part of hospice is (1.0) for the most part you get
3 to do whatever you ↓want. (0.5) hh ((chuckles)) (0.5)
4 FM: That ↑don't sound too ↑bad. ((chuckles))
5 MD: (0.2) There's not much people saying well >we can't do this for you because
6 it's going to make it harder to do this. For the most part people say<
7 whatever makes you comfortable, (0.2) We'll try to make it happen. (1.2)
8 People (0.8) come see you on a regular basis whether it's at ↑home or in
9 the hospital or in- not the hospital but (0.2) >an inpatient setting like a
10 hospice<(0.5) ↑home.
11 Pt: Right. (0.2)
12 MD: >There would be people who are always following ↑you< who are (.)
13 closely watching (.) how your symptoms are managed to >make sure that
14 your ↑pain is managed< your >shortness of ↑breath is managed< And
15 you're as ↑comfortable as we can make you.
16 Pt: Is there somebody there like 24 hours? =No?
17 MD: At home? =No. [At ↑home (.) ↑no.]
18 Pt: Oh okay   [I didn't WANT THAT.] (0.8)
19 MD: °No.° (0.5)
20 MD2: In fact that's an important thing to know about.=↑If you wanted to
21 learn more about ↓this (0.8) then we would ask one of the hospice
22 providers

The series of continuers and confirmations in lines 4 to 22 on the patient's part builds an interactional momentum that prompts the family member in line 4 to affiliate with the patient's assents, asking what we see as one of the most common unprompted questions that family members tend to have in end-of-life settings where Palliative Care approaches are being favored: namely, will the patient be able to eat and drink. The patient's clarification in line 18 that she was not disappointed by the physician's answer in line 17 appears to be designed to maintain the positive solidarity the group has developed around the idea of hospice as a logical choice for her. What we notice, generally, from this conversation is that getting patients and family members to actively query Palliative Care in a detailed way often requires a preparatory sequential environment characterized by continuers and intensive signals of alignment, which together create a preference for specific follow-up questions. Without these interactional features, patients and family members may pose no questions at all.

For **concerns about eating and drinking**, see 8.4, 10.10. For **characterizations of hospice**, see 10.12, 4.5, 5.5.

3.7 Insights and implications from Chapter 3

What we hope to have shown in this chapter is one spectrum of ways families, patients, and clinicians clear interactional ground for questioning Palliative Care – whether from a social, ritual, interactional, moral, philosophical, or procedural point of view. Family-initiated characterizations and portrayals, derived from previous experiences of others' illnesses, appear to be an important resource for a successful Palliative Care consultation, and the general availability of this resource will grow in the US as the years go on. In conversation 3.2, we saw an instance in which a seriously-ill patient had little experience with palliative modalities beyond a family experience that had been negative and morally troubling for her. Palliative Care consultations today can do double duty, in the sense that they can provide comfort to seriously-ill persons while also alleviating long-held and often shame-inducing worries about difficult deaths in their families' pasts. This micro-historical aspect is, of course, an important component of holistic wellness in the present. We also have asked what conditions, circumstances, and stances on the part of the clinician may tend to preclude such questions, whether for epistemic, stylistic, or ideological reasons. In the next chapter, we turn to the ways in which patients disclose their identities and desires to clinicians. Chapter Four closes Part One on Introductions and Presentations.

4 Presenting the self

The foregoing chapters presented a spectrum of interactions in which clinicians (re-)presented Palliative Care as a medical specialty to patients and families (Chapter Two) and where patients queried, questioned, challenged, and sought information about Palliative Care (Chapter Three) through various interventions of their own. While the conversations presented in those two chapters included substantive and meaningful moments in which patients foregrounded their identities, selves, and preferred self-characterizations amid other topics at hand, this current chapter emphasizes such moments primarily. We will remember in conversation 2.1, for instance, that the patient styled himself the "silent partner" in the ensuing Palliative Care consultation and yet, three turns later, reclaimed the floor in an anything but silent fashion. In conversation 2.2, the patient stylized herself as an exacerbated provider who indulges the unpredictable needs of hospital personnel. In 3.2, it was important for the patient to be recognized as a daughter, who had once cared for a dying father. In 3.3, the patient's vocation as a volunteer hospice chaplain remained unacknowledged in the initial portion of the consultation, which led to some awkward clinician-initiated repair halfway through. The son-in-law in 3.5 is proud of his creative formulations as a spokesperson for the benefits of hospice care, joking that he wants to copyright his metaphor about hospice services as an adaptively "amoebous blob." Each of these persons wishes to be recognized and remembered in these ways, and their contributions to these complex interactions are designed accordingly. Such emerging designs in interaction – knitting together a sensible portrayal of one's historical self, one's facework in the current moment, amid the contingencies of the hospital context – are the focus of the following series of conversations.

4.1 We're not deep thinkers

The prospect of a medical specialty whose 'procedure' involves not traditional surgical and pharmacological interventions but rather the procedures of conversation, reflection, coordination, and goals-of-care planning can be linguistically daunting. Particularly for those who may, for good reason, mistrust institutional language or are disinclined to lay claim to language rights when it comes to clinically complex matters. Wishing to have their disease or symptoms addressed with traditional curative treatment, rather than with talk – i.e., with actions, rather than words – many patients and families in the hospital would rather forego conversation (with strangers) altogether, if they could. What's more, the presumed

https://doi.org/10.1515/9781501504570-004

profundity or immensity of the topic of dying is not a welcome prospect for conversational exploration for many, who might just as well prefer to handle dying in
the pragmatic, no-nonsense, or sleeping-dogs-lie fashion they may have handled
other problems throughout their lives. The suggestion that dying well might
require a different kind of preparatory talk that is challenging, uncomfortable,
and unhabitual – and that such talk is proper to the hospital context as much
as it is proper to, say, spiritual and religious traditions – elicits eagerness and
relief for some, resistance and perplexity for others. Conversation 4.1 introduces
a patient who imagines a group-level identity called "deep thinkers" who ponder
spiritual and existential questions about mortality – and insists that he (and his
spouse) are not among them.

The following conversation prompts us to consider these questions:
1) Does the Palliative Care consultation genre tend to elicit certain responses
   and self-characterizations as to patients' and families' *general* inclinations
   towards talking and collaborative thinking?
2) Are such identities around exploratory conversation framed as individual
   and/or collective attributes and preferences?
3) What kinds of topics and prompts evoke the (welcome or unwelcome) prospect of "deep thinking"?
4) How do patients and families design identities in interaction that help position
   them advantageously vis-à-vis other emerging projects in the conversation?

The patient in the following conversation self-identifies as an 85-year-old white
man and as financially secure, reporting graduate-level education and Christian
religious affiliation. He has been diagnosed with a stage-four prostate cancer. He
believes he is "very likely" to live for a year, while his clinician-rated survival
prognosis at the time of the following consultation is six months. In fact, he lived
78 days beyond this consultation, i.e., shorter than both the clinical expectation
and his own. The patient strongly ranks his end-of-life goals as "comfort over
longevity," and he rates his "global" quality-of-life over the previous two days
at a six out of ten. The following portion of talk occurred during the first visit
of the Palliative Care team. The clinicians speaking in the conversation are a
Palliative Care physician and a PC nurse practitioner. The group is talking about
the patient's current discharge plan, as previously described by an absent clinician of another specialty, probably an oncologist. The Palliative Care physician
asks the group what they are expecting when he is discharged:

1 Sp: Straight home, having some re<u>hab,</u> but he says ↑he <u>thinks</u> he could come
2   straight ↓home.
3 Pt: [↑I think   ]

 4 MD: [↑↑The >physical] therapist will be able to weigh in on that as well.<
 5 NP: Right.
 6 Pt: Yeah, >but the physical therapists over there are good and<
 7   [and one of them are good friends.] but
 8 NP: [↑Here (.) Here are you working] working,
 9 Pt: No.
10 NP: ↑Here are you ↑working with the physical ther:apist?
11 Pt: Yeah.
12 NP: You are?
13 MD: THEY HAVE YOU DO EXER↑CISES?
14 NP: Cause- cause they are also able to <u>assess</u>:-
15 Sp: Uh huh.
16 NP: Like (.) <u>do</u> they f:eel: you're- that's what >they're <u>good</u> at,<
17   [are you physi]cally ready to go ho:me?
18 Pt: [Yeah, I'm I'm]
19 NP: [or re:hab]
20 Sp: [As he said, I'm 85] and I can't take ↑care of him, but
21   (.) I mean he's a big guy.
22 NP: So we'll depend on- on- on the physical therapist to- to help us <u>assess</u>
23   your (.) your capabi↓lity.

We display this initial section because it clarifies how various participants in
the talk are creating allyship with one another around two competing projects
for pre-discharge. The clinician-led project, supported by the patient's spouse
who aligns with it implicitly later, in line 20, is to establish a sensibility of consensus around the notion that the in-house physical therapists should stop by
prior to discharge to assess whether the patient is in good enough form to return
home, a goal that the physician is strenuously pursuing. In lines 6–7, the patient
recruits to his current project the competing credibility of absent physical therapists "over there", i.e., in a district closer to his home, thereby undermining the
physician's contention in line 4 that he may not simply be able to "come straight
home." Being able to go home is often an intensely cherished vision and ideal
for patients in Palliative Care consultations, and many patients experience clinicians' skepticism about the details of this "going home" as a threat to be handled
adversarially.

By characterizing the prospective role of an on-site physical therapy team
in discharge planning with the positively connotated phrases "will be able to
weigh in on that," "as well", and "are good at", the physician tips off the patient
to his own developing project: that there should not be a discharge "straight
home" without express support of the in-house physical therapist. This threat

toward the patient's negative face then escalates, as (in lines 8, 10, 12, and 13) the nurse practitioner and physician ask and then seek confirmation from the patient about the extent of his involvement in in-hospital physical therapy currently. Lines 14 and 16 then begin a face-developing sequence valorizing the (absent) in-house physical therapists, and this project is also simultaneously expressive of a continuing disalignment with the patient's project of "going straight home."

Meanwhile, the spouse's disfluency in line 20–21 ("but (.) I mean") indicates her ambivalence, but ultimate alignment, with the clinicians' project of recruiting approval for the plan to see physical therapy for an assessment prior to hospital discharge. It takes until line 22 for the nurse practitioner, emboldened by the patient's spouse's outright statement that "I can't take care of him" physically, due to his size, to foreclose the topic with the phrase "We'll depend on." This future-tense formulation blends intention with prediction so as to avert the impression of constraining the patient's autonomy. The focus in this sequence is thus on investing in the competence, status, and indispensability of the non-present physical therapy team, and this campaign will lead the patient to re-seize the floor (below) and thus the prerogative to promote his own face, displacing the currently emerging solidarity frame. Noting these dynamics coalescing to his disadvantage, the patient seizes the floor for a troubles-telling that he had first attempted to begin in line 18 above. He shifts the focus from his current readiness and capacity to return home to a reassertion of his enduring identity as a "strong" person.

1 Pt: I'm <u>actually</u> very strong (0.5) I subdued 26 <u>people</u> the other night. hhh (0.5)
2 NP: T-hh!
3 MD: Uhh. (1.0)
4 NP: WHAT ↑HAPPENED?
5 Pt: Hallucination.
6 NP: <Oh: boy.>
7 MD: AP↑PARENTLY.
8 Pt: Gave me too many steroids and I-
9 Sp: injured a ↑nurse? ((laugh))
10 NP: <Oh no. hhh>
11 MD: ↓Aw.
12 Pt: Then they tried, they tried to hold me down and,
13 MD: He thought it-
14 NP: No it <u>wasn't</u> your fault.
15 Sp: No and he wasn't physical,
16 MD: I'M <u>GLAD</u> YOU'RE feeling be↓tter.

17 Sp: He's a gen<u>tle</u> man.
18 Pt: [Still] hundred percent.
19 NP: [I can], I can see that. I can see that.

This is an example of a patient strategically reversing the frame of the talk by way of an identity-telling that insulates him against the kind of interactional opposition he had just been experiencing. "Strength" being of incontrovertible value in a setting of serious illness, he is able to regain the upper-hand with a story framed around it, and around the 'good news' announcement that he is "actually" stronger than expected. The preceding talk, about the (absent) in-house physical therapists' abilities – as well as the clinicians' non-acknowledgement of the patients' assessment of his physical therapists back home (in line 6 on page 93 above), the euphemistic implicature in line 4 on page 93 that in-house physical therapy will need to approve his discharge, and the round of skeptical confirmatory questioning about the extent of the patient's involvement in in-house PT – combine to prompt the patient to engage what we might (drawing on political vernacular) call the "nuclear option." Namely, the patient successfully clears the floor of all of the above negotiations, albeit temporarily, with a telling about his own strength and potential for unintentional force and violence, which is a repertoire he prefers to thematize over thought-and-planning-heavy topics like assessment and preparedness for discharge. Strength trumps coordination of care.

Using the word "subdued" in line 1 allows the patient to tell a story of his superhuman strength, manifested (in his view) by hospital staff having given him too many steroids, thus providing one more implicit reason for an undelayed discharge. No overadministering of sterroids, no subduing of people. The long pauses in line 1 above indicate that his story has indeed shifted the frame of the interaction so much that the other participants are taken aback, which is confirmed in lines 2 and 3 by both the nurse practitioner and Palliative Care physician coming out of face briefly with a snicker-like token and a grunt, respectively. It is not clear if these are continuers, response tokens, or outcries, but the nurse practitioner recovers with a response in line 4 that befits concern about an unfortunate outcome, rather than a celebrating a person's self-assessment of strength. Nonetheless, the patient's project to regain the floor and to accomplish positive face accrual for himself is quite successful in lines 12–19, which double as repair for the recounted, unintended expression of violence/strength and as an occasion to solicit a positive characterization of the patient.

This is a complex moment because it displays the often-constrained terms by which seriously-ill patients are able to obtain acknowledgement for the characteristics of historical self they hold most valuable. Physical strength in the present (not in his past) is a trait the patient puts out for appreciation, at a moment when the conversation is primarily geared toward driving toward consensus about the superordinate capacities of a non-present party and about the imprudence of "going straight home." This is not a mere self-aggrandizing outburst from the patient, but rather an attempt to reestablish equilibrium as to which aspects of (his) self are or ought to be most valued in the current interaction. The clinicians' strongly disprefer any acknowledgement of the patient's strength, assuaging with ascriptions of gentleness and faultlessness. The patient continues by upping the ante on his self-styled exceptionalism:

1 Pt: >It's too bad you're taking up room with me<. I should be out with the (.)
2   boys (.) raking <u>leaves</u>. =↑Something (.) anything (1.2) But ↑this is <u>easy</u>.
3 MD: Sir, what else can we <u>help</u> you with <u>today</u>?
4 Pt: ↑Right now? we- we're not ↑deep thinkers at this point, I think.
5 Sp: °What did he ↑↑say?°
6 NP: We're <u>not</u> deep thinkers. hh um (.) and.
7 Pt: I, I think, we, ↑we've covered pretty (.) pretty good?
8 NP: And- and <u>you</u> feel that you're- you're- your l:evel of <u>pain</u> control:
9   right now is: <u>go:</u>od?
10 Pt: ↑Really haven't <u>had</u> >that much <u>pain</u>.<

The implicature in line 1–4 is rich with several phenomena. The Palliative Care physician takes the patient's preferred near-term outcome, about being "out raking leaves with the boys" and his characterization of hospitalization as "This is easy", as an indication that it is time to close the consultation, by eliciting (but not necessarily encouraging) any further topics. He addresses the patient as "sir", thus reinstating the level of formality appropriate to conversation openings and closings. The patient's response to this pre-closing is an identity statement about "we", i.e. he and his wife, which implies that the sort of topic or help offered by the Palliative Care team is *deep thinking*. Only two turns earlier, the patient himself was indeed engaged in a form of what could easily be considered deep thought, as he is reminiscing about raking leaves, and being with the boys (Drew and Holt 1998b). But this kind of deep thinking did not find uptake from the Palliative Care clinicians, who understood it as a resistance to, rather than an engagement in, topics of relevance to the care.

For **expressions about going home**, see *10.12, 4.5, 5.4*. For **characterizations of a patient's strength**, see *3.4, 9.3, 9.1, 5.5*. For **images of the outdoors**, see *3.1, 5.4*. For characterizations of serious illness as **hard or easy**, see *7.5, 9.4, 4.3, 4.2*.

4.2 You're a survivor

The previous conversation features a situation in which a patient strategically derails the clinicians' project by interjecting an extraordinary story about his own physical strength. In conversation 4.2, which involves only two people (patient and clinician), the patient is engaged in a project of telling a story about his overall disposition toward illness, which might be summarized as (what the patient sees as) a puzzling resilience over the course of a life in which "my body's been fighting forever" (in line 6 on page 100 below). Meanwhile, however, the clinician is going through a series of questionnaire questions that conflict interactionally with the telling of a holistic story. The way these two frames conflict is evident in how the clinician responds to, affiliates with, or aligns with the emerging story the patient is telling over the course of the questionnaire-taking. The questions we pose at the outset, then, are:

1) How do patients' self-characterization in narrative conflict interactionally with the genre of the questionnaire, and what are the ramifications of this conflict (see Antaki et al. 1996)?

2) How, and for what interactional purposes, do patients invest in stories of their own surprising resilience?

The patient in the following conversation self-identifies as a 54-year-old white man and as financially secure, reporting Associate's-level education and Christian religious affiliation. He has been diagnosed with a stage-four colon cancer. He believes he is unable to estimate his prognosis, while his clinician-rated survival prognosis at the time of the following consultation is three to six months. In fact, he lived eight days beyond this consultation, i.e., drastically shorter than clinically expected. The patient strongly ranks his end-of-life goals as "comfort over longevity," and he rates his "global" quality-of-life over the previous two days – i.e., physical, emotional, social, spiritual, and financial quality – at an eight out of ten. The following portion of talk occurred during the first visit of the Palliative Care team, and the clinician speaking is a Palliative Care nurse practitioner. The patient is giving a summary of the ubiquity of illness in the experiences of his siblings and other family members over the course of their lives:

1 Pt: Because we've all been, uh- I mean (.) we've all been pretty <u>sick</u>=Uh even my
2   little <u>sister</u>=Like I said I had (.) meningitis (.) and my sister caught the same
3   thing and she went deaf °↓from it.°
4 NP: ↑Wow.
5 Pt: And ↑she was even worse than <u>me</u> when I was- when ↑she was young so.
6   ((coughs))

7 NP: So, hh (.) you're un<u>emp</u>loyed right now?

8 Pt: Uh, I'm (.) <u>dis</u>abled.

9 NP: Disabled.

10 Pt: Yes.

11 NP: Um, what were- what did you used to do (.) I mean,

12   [when we ↑talked about the:]

13 Pt: [I was a carpenter].

14 NP: Uh- okay=I figured it was something with

15   [construction or °something° with ↑glass.]

16 Pt: [Yeah, I was a carpenter most of my   ]   life, but (.) I did carpentry

17   and worked in ↑restaurants: and (.) <u>what</u>ever ↓else.

18 NP: °Yeah.°

19 Pt: So (.) I probably had like three or four jobs in my whole life.

20 NP: ↓Yeah.

21 Pt: In 30, 40 years.

22 NP: ↑Nice. °↓Yeah.°

We note that the clinician does not, in line 9, inquire about the nature of the patient's self-described disability, which itself was a correction of her confirmatory question whether he was unemployed. From line 11–12, the clinician continues to pursue her question about employment (rather than discussing disability), and appears to have corrected her incipient formulation "what were- [you before you were disabled]" with a question formulated more typically for those who are retired, "what did you used to do?" (We will remember that this patient is 54 years old and thus on the low end of the presumptive retirement age.) The patient accommodates the clinician's request for vocational information, but he narrativizes his vocational history extensively, at first foregrounding a diversity of employment in lines 16 and 17 but then sharply correcting this impression of jack-of-all-trades identity with the morally coded assertion in line 19 and 21 that he does not *jump from job to job*. These are complex self-characterizations, but as Antaki, Houtkoop-Steenstra, and Rapley (2000: 236) have demonstrated, the clinician's interview frame makes it difficult for clinicians to engage in much substantive acknowledgement or alignment, and this clinician indeed primarily responds to his story with "a (permissive) sequence of [answer receipt] + [right/ok token] + [high-grade assessment] + [move to next item]" (ibid.). Were the clinician's response in line 22 to be taken as substantive and not interview-framed, the clinician would essentially be promoting the patient's moral claim that fewer jobs make for a more valorous work history. But it does not appear such a moral assent is implicated, so much as the desire to move through the questionnaire without delay. In line 14, the clinician does indeed affiliate with the patient by showing that she previously "figured" he had worked in one industry rather than another, but this is the single show of epistemic alignment with his contributions. The clinician then offers a provisional summary:

```
1   Pt:   So. .hhhhh ((coughs)) (2.0)
2   NP:   ↑So hhh sounds like this is really kind of a rough spot and- and=I guess,
3         in summary=I guess what I'm hearing is that (.) it's um: (1.4) we really
4         need to have some clarification: a little bit more about your disease from
5         Dr. ____ and ____.
6   Pt:   Well, ↑they've come in and told me about ↓that, you know =he said it's
7         (1.0) like I said- he said it's ↓spreading and he hasn't given me a ↑time
8         date but-
9   NP:   Okay.
10  Pt:   The way he's talked (.) I'd (1.0) basically, I'm looking maybe at (.) it
11        could be anywhere from (.) to↑day (1.5) >maybe seven to eight months
12        down the road. Maybe< two ↑years? pro↓bably.
13  NP:   And-
14  Pt:   It all depends what they feel like they want to ↑do and (0.5) since I (0.5)
15        ↑basically: (.) nobody knows what they want to ↓do with me now.
16  NP:   Yeah, as far as treat↓ments.
17  Pt:   Yes.
18  NP:   And that's what I hear you needing to have more information about.
19  Pt:   Y:eah=That's what I'm wai↓ting for because, uh =he said (.) he was just
20        going to throw in the ↓towel.
21  NP:   °Okay.°
```

What emerges in this string of talk is a competitive framing (Goffman 1974), in which the patient bids to characterize his prognosis as dependent on (non-present) clinicians' relative willingness to pursue further curative / invasive treatment. In line 10, the patient foregrounds "the way he's [the oncologist] talked" as the primary resource for his own coming to understand the relationship between his prognosis and clinicians' willingness. Throughout this assessment, the Palliative Care clinician employs the therapeutic recasting phrase "I guess what I'm hearing is that" (line 3) and "that's what I'm hearing you needing" (line 18) regarding the prospect of ascertaining an absent clinician's intentions. But she does not go so far as to acknowledge that the patient is describing a predicament in which his longevity appears to be dependent on various clinicians' willingness to not give up on him, an assessment he has reached inferentially by way of how they, "the oncologists," talk. Without aligning or disaligning with his analysis, the clinician recasts his contribution as a request for *more information* in line 18. The patient's requested confirmatory response is complex, beginning with "Yeah, that's what I'm waiting for" but continuing with a disjunctive focus not on information but on the questionable legitimacy of the information the patient had already been given. Rather than *his* need for more information, the clinician might have formulated it as her own, or her team's own need for more information from the oncologists. This is of course a difficult interdisciplinary clinical dilemma, because Palliative Care specialists are often the primary interpreters of vagary or nondisclosure in the language of oncologists, as they make their prognostic assessments about individual patients they are referring for a Palliative Care consultation.

We could imagine that another version of this conversation could have included patient statements like "I find it unacceptable that" or "I'm angry/confused that" the oncologist appears to have "thrown in the towel," but this patient does not select such adversarial formulations, choosing to accommodate, align, and then subtly disalign with the status quo of communication with his oncologists. Yet his disalignments receive no uptake from the Palliative Care clinician here, which leads the patient to frame the situation as an abnormal mystery of sorts:

1	Pt:	And that's why they can't under<u>stand</u> it? So-
2	NP:	Okay. (1.2)
3	Pt:	I'm throwing them all for a loop and they're like wondering what's going
4		↑on with <u>this</u> ↓guy.
5	NP:	Yeah. (1.5)
6	Pt:	My body's been fighting forever.
7	NP:	Yeah (.) Weird =You're a- you're a sur<u>vi</u>vor?
8	Pt:	↑I gotta do <u>some</u>thing?
9	NP:	Yeah.
10	Pt:	If I didn't sur<u>vive</u>? I wouldn't be here?
11	NP:	Are you um- I'm just gonna run through a few little other questions?
12	Pt:	Oh no go ahead!
13	NP:	Are you- are you- you feel ↑tired?
14	Pt:	↑Um ↑actually, I feel a little <u>tired</u>, only °because of the medica↓tion
15		and stuff and-°
16	NP:	↑Okay=And- and you're <u>not</u> having any nausea <u>now</u>?
17	Pt:	No. No.
18	NP:	°Okay.°
19	Pt:	°No.°
20	NP:	And um, any ↑pai:n?
21	Pt:	I di- um <u>no</u>. it's just uncomfortableness,

The reason why this conversation is included here, rather than say in Chapter Ten on prognosis, or in Chapter Seven on absent others, is that the project underlying the patients' disalignments, which are consistently dispreferred by the clinician, is to characterize himself as a life-long fighter of disease – and not only that, but a member of a family of life-long fighters against disease. This charismatically told story prepares the way for a meritocratic sense for why his oncologists should continue aggressively treating his colon cancer – not because that's what he expressly *wants*, but because of the kind of person he *is*. The development of this project conflicts, however, with the questionnaire genre currently being performed by the clinician. In line 7, the clinician does indeed find herself compelled to affiliate with the patient's self-characterization as someone whose "body's been fighting forever," and she does so through the reformulation "You're a survivor," which has a summative, expeditive function here rather than an affiliative one (on survivor metaphors, see Appleton and Flynn 2014; Gill 1998). This summative identity-formulation allows the clinician to continue the questionnaire unimpeded. The question we are left with is whether questionnaire-taking in this setting necessarily requires such expeditive formulations and neutral-stance acknowledgements, or whether the work of information-gathering can proceed in a way that does not tend to overlook complex narrative contributions and analyses on the part of the patient.

The patient is clearly eager to project an integrated life story predicated on surprising accomplishments and mysterious resilience. Noteworthy here is that the patient lived for only eight more days after this consultation, and likely spent the last days of his life in drastic "prognostic discordance" with his clinical team (Gramling et al. 2017; see also Horne et al. 2005; Jones and Beach 2005). This raises the question whether the nurse practitioner's affirmative recasting throughout this conversation furthered this discordance, and whether taking a more assertive approach may have benefited the patient in some way. We note that throughout the conversation, the nurse practitioner does relatively little of the talking, allowing the patient to weave a web of stories and anecdotes that portray him as someone who stumps the oncologists who, he reports, are inclined to "throw in the towel."

For **expressions of surprising resilience and survivorship**, see 7.5, 9.4, 4.3, 4.1.

4.3 What I really want is peace

We have presented some interactions (2.1 and 4.2 for instance) in which patients are successfully able to style themselves as central and authoritative, even when they seem to distribute primary speaking privileges to others. Some may see in such interactions an aura of "holding court" or the like, and this designed centrality necessarily intersects with other forms of speaker privilege, including age, gender, and familial status. The following is another such conversation in which the patient uses certain interactional techniques to establish himself in a privileged position of speakership throughout the conversation, which allows him to manage topics and leave-takings in powerful ways. Our question is thus: what are some techniques that enable seriously-ill patients to establish the prerogative to hold the floor and to determine both topics and the proper treatment of those topics?

The patient in the following conversation self-identifies as a 63-year-old Black man and as financially insecure, reporting Bachelor's-level education and Muslim religious affiliation. He has been diagnosed with a stage-four kidney cancer. He believes he is "very likely" to live for a year, while his clinician-rated survival prognosis at the time of the following consultation is two weeks to three months. In fact, he lived 135 days beyond this consultation, i.e., longer than clinically expected, but much shorter than he himself expected. The patient strongly ranks his end-of-life goals as "comfort over longevity," and he rates his "global" quality-of-life over the previous two days at a five out of ten. The following portion of talk occurred during the second visit of the Palliative Care team. The clinicians speaking are two PC nurse practitioners, and the clinician-initiated topic is "what is bothering you the most":

1	Pt:	So what's ↑bothering me the <u>most</u> is ↓uh (1.5) uh:: uh:::: ((laughter))
2	Fr:	(laughing) He's laughing
3	FM:	Where to <u>start</u>,
4	Pt:	This guy here.
5	NP:	That guy here he's ↑bothering you the most?
6	Pt:	Yeah that guy's bothering me the most. (0.2) He he won't leave?
7	Fr:	((laughter))
8	NP:	Oh yeah?
9	Pt:	Huh uh.
10	NP:	He's at:tached to you:.
11	Pt:	Yeah. =He's here like 24 hours a <u>day</u> even but I'll ↑have this <u>establishment</u>
12		throw him out.
13	Fr:	((laughter))
14	Pt:	He says I've been thrown out of better es↑tablishments than ↓this.
15	NP:	((laughter)) hhh
16	Pt:	Uh (0.8) but uh (0.5) ↑no uh (1.2) what bothers me the most pro↓bably is to.
17		Worry about. To think about those people that I care about.
18	NP:	Sure.

19 NP2: ( ) the uncertainty of what's going to come forward
20 Pt: Yeah. I think that's what's uh (1.0) that's] what ↓bothers me.

Prior to this section, the patient had been asked to share what is bothering him the most in the hospital and in his illness at the moment. Beginning to answer the question, he notices a family friend entering the room and pivots from the answer he is about to formulate and gives as a temporary stand-in answer "this guy here" as what's bothering him the most. The spontaneous self-entitlement to reframe the question to incorporate a light-hearted joke at the expense of a newly joined member of the talk continues in lines 11–14. The patient frames his hospital room or, metonymically, the entire hospital as "this establishment," thus re-styling it as a place of public social encounter, such as a restaurant, a café, or other service-sector business, in which there are wanted and unwanted "characters" and rules of hospitality and decorum. This is a powerful metonymy, because it consolidates for the patient the symbolic prerogative to 1) generously confer and qualify membership, and 2) determine, or hold sway over, the conduct in "this establishment."

Having completed the joke, the patient then issues a 'but-seriously' pivot in line 16 and waits for the laughter to subside. He then is able to continue to formulate his answer to the question initially posed, in which the family friend teased in the previous turns is implicitly re-invited into the fold of "those people that I care about." This topic of concern to the patient resurfaces at the end of the consultation:

1 NP: We're almost done. Are there any ↑things >I haven't asked you about that
2 you want to make <u>sure</u> I focus on. <We talked about the pai:n and some of
3 the other symptoms= °I can try and make some recommendations°.
4 Pt: Well the last- The thing I really want you to focus on now is my religion
5 ((laughter))
6 NP: Okay.
7 Pt: And that's the ↑last thing we talked about.
8 NP: I know=I didn't want to interrupt.
9 Pt: ((laughter))
10 NP: Um. (0.5) But <u>t</u>ell me what you want. (1.0)
11 Pt: What I <u>want</u> is peace:.
12 NP: °Mm-hmm.°
13 Pt: And what I want is peace (0.5) peace for myself, but more importantly
14 for my ↓friends.
15 NP: °Mm-hmm.°

The patient seizes the occasion of the clinician's pre-closing in lines 1–3 above to reassert his prerogative to set the order of priorities and values in the conversation, a prerogative that Palliative Care consultations typically seek to encourage under the rubric of "goals-of-care" and "quality-of-life" discussions. In lines 11–13 above the patient recycles the clinician's phrase "what you want" to open a preamble to the following existential vision of the future:

```
 1 Pt:   I want that all of my friends (1.2) the: experience the:: (1.2) joy and
 2       pleasure of being a Mus↓lim (0.5) And I know, everybody from (0.5)
 3       every religion could probably say that.
 4 NP:   °Mm-hmm.°
 5 Pt:   And with some (0.8) conviction.
 6 NP:   °Mm-hmm.°
 7 Pt:   You know, but at the same time (0.8) uh, I reached a point in my ↑life
 8       where it's (0.8) a choice ↓of (0.8) how much do you think about (1.4) your
 9       ↑life as being (0.8) life (0.5) as we're doing right now, breathing?
10 NP:   °Mm-hmm?°
11 Pt:   And inter↑acting with each other↑ and all that, (0.8) Or life as: (1.2) as the
12       com↑plete (0.5) aspect of ↓life (0.5) when you're not ↓breathing.
13 NP:   °Mm-hmm,°
14 Pt:   When you're not uh:: (2.8) at a point where: you need to have uh::
15       (0.5) oxygen and-
16 NP:   °Mm-hmm.° (1.8)
17 Pt:   And ↑metals: and (.) chemicals and all that stuff=
18 NP:   =Physical body.
19 Pt:   ↑Yeah=you don't need that °anymore.°
20 NP:   Right.
```

The patient seems to have fully accepted the holistic premises of the Palliative Care consultation and its contemplative, practical focus on a wide range of quality-of-life deliberations in the context of serious illness, while the clinician in line 1–3 on page 103 is prepared to summarize the outcomes of the conversation as primarily symptom- and pain-management oriented. Put another way, the "can of worms" that the Palliative Care consultation discussion has prompted for the patient appears to be welcome and inspiring, such that he wishes to somewhat spontaneously explore existential questions about joy, peace, the finitude of human life, and the "complete aspect of life" in death or the afterlife. We noted in conversation 4.1 that, in the same sequential environment as the patient claimed that "we're not deep thinkers," he was nonetheless wistfully invoking "raking leaves with the boys." (On timing, see Auer et al. 1999; Bilmes 1985; see also Jefferson 1973.) There is, in these conversations, often a subtle and deceptive proximity, sequentially speaking, between "deep thought" as the speaker in 4.1 characterized it, and the ostensive refusal of it. How can Palliative Care continue to expand the number and diversity of paths that seriously-ill patients have available to them to express their current orientation toward values like joy, peace, "the complete aspect of life" and other spontaneous cosmological formulations – even and especially when they are suffering symptoms that constrain other aspects of their quality-of-life?

For **religious reflections,** *see 4.3. For* **existential and philosophical reflec-tions on life and death,** *see 3.2, 6.2, 4.4, 6.2, 6.4.*

4.4 But there could always be a magical thing

Sometimes the primary situated identity patients invest in most in these con-versations is precisely that of the "exception to the rule," who – in the face of a decidedly negative prognostic forecast – is all the more committed to being the one who overcomes odds, with or without divine, supernatural, or human help. The question we pose in this conversation is: can Palliative Care clinicians have a meaningful and supportive interaction with seriously-ill patients who insist they are the exceptional kind of person who beats the odds, whatever the odds are – even when clinical prognosis will lead to prognostic discordance with the patient?

The patient in the following conversation self-identifies as a 66-year-old white woman and as financially secure, reporting Associate's-level education and Christian religious affiliation. She has been diagnosed with stage-four lung cancer. She believes she will live for another year at least, while her clinician-rated survival prognosis at the time of the following consultation is two weeks to three months. In fact, she lived 11 days beyond this date, drastically shorter than her own expectations and nominally shorter than the clinicians' expectations. The patient is unsure whether she prefers pursuing care focused on comfort or lon-gevity, and she rates her "global" quality-of-life over the previous two days – i.e., physical, emotional, social, spiritual, and financial quality – at a three out of ten. The following portion of talk occurred during the first visit of the Palliative Care team. The clinician speaking is a medical resident training in Palliative Care. Referring to the patient's chart, the resident is recapping what another physician had spoken about with the patient regarding options for hospice care.

1 Res: Right and he had mentioned <u>hos</u>pice and you sss (.) expressed a lot of
2   int<u>erest</u> in <u>tha:t</u> and the ability to go <u>home</u> (0.8) and (.) and be
3   ↑comfortable ↓there. (1.2) Is that- (.) am I am
4   [.... I remembering that correctly?]

5 Pt: [Well I <u>figure</u> that you're better] comfortable over you
6   ((clearing throat)) own situation in your own (0.2) <u>hou:se</u> (0.8) and
7   your own things:. (0.5)
8 Res: Is that (.) pr↑actical though or–
9 Pt: And my [<u>family</u>.]
10 Res: [at this point or]
11 Pt: <They could come and go as they <u>plea:se</u>.> (0.2)
12 Res: There's just one more step to all that because um (0.2) >you and I discussed
13   a little bit more about what <u>hospice</u>< en:↑<u>tails</u> this mor↓ning. (0.5) And
14   then you said to me (.) >several times< (.) I'm not going to die. >I'm going
15   to ↑live.< (1.5) Um so we wanted to sort of (0.5) <u>help</u> (1.0) clarify for
16   everybody <u>here:</u> (0.2) sort of (0.5) what (0.2) what those two things mean
17   because (0.5) <u>hospice</u> >like I said this morning is sort of-< it's almost a
18   phi↑losophy not- >it's not just a <u>pla:ce</u>.<
19 Pt: Yeah.
20 Res: It's actually a <u>way</u> of trying to ap<u>proach</u> your <u>ill</u>↓ness (0.5) that isn't
21   (0.8) com↑<u>pletely</u> in line with what you're saying >what you also said<
22   (0.5) which (.) that you wanted to be <u>pretty</u> ag<u>gre</u>ssive with how you
23   >↑treat a thing< because you said (.) I'm <u>not</u> gonna let this (1.0) end my
24   life, =I'm gonna (0.2) I'm gonna ↑beat <u>this</u>. (0.2) And those two things
25   don't really match ↑<u>up</u>. (1.0) Um I know Dr. ____' s↑poke with ↓you -
26 Pt: °<u>Right</u>. °
27 Res: And did that (0.2) sort of change your thinking?

This is an important example of a Palliative Care clinician seeking, in as accurate
terms as possible, to recognize a patient's emphatic desire to pursue aggressive
curative treatment despite available prognostic indications otherwise. Here the
medical resident, in training for specialization in Palliative Care, is reasoning
with the patient not about her prognosis per se, but about the logic of beating the
odds of stage-four lung cancer while also availing oneself of hospice resources.
In lines 5–6, the patient indicates that her understanding of hospice is primarily
that it is tantamount to being comfortable. The medical resident, perhaps for the
sake of audience-design in the larger group setting, phrases his nonalignment
euphemistically, suggesting that hospice is "not completely in line with what
you're saying." In the following section, the mentoring attending Palliative Care
physician takes the floor and seeks to develop with the patient a re-analysis of her
perceived relationship between hospice and her comfort.

1 Pt: They. know. my. way. (0.2)
2 MD: Did that- did[speaking with them change=

 3 Pt: =No.
 4 MD: =your thinking about what you're fee<u>ling:</u>?
 5 Pt: Nope. (1.2) His job tonight is to go <u>home</u> and dream? (1.2) <that God to go in
 6   his little <u>brain</u>> (0.5) make a little micro<u>tape</u> (1.2) come out of that dream (.)
 7   play that microtape >which is gonna ↓help fix ↓me.< ((laughter)) (0.8)
 8   It's the <u>job</u> I gave ↓him. (0.2)
 9 Res: You gave him a job to ↑<u>fix you</u>,
10 Pt: [Yeah.]
11 FM: [Yeah.] (0.8)
12 FM: °That's his job for the night.° ((laughter))
13 Pt: Do you see where I'm <u>that</u> (1.2) <u>optimis</u>↓ti- You ↓know. (1.0)

In line 25 on page 106, the resident has referred to an oncologist the patient knows
well and asked whether he may have suggested she reconsider the reconcilability
of enrolling in hospice with her "beat the odds" stance. In response, she reas-
suredly states in line 1 on page 106 that oncology "know my way," a way she will
elaborate upon in subsequent turns. She then tells of having given the oncologist
a task to communicate through his dreams to God, who will then direct his treatment of her toward ultimate success – i.e., remission of the cancer. The metaphor
of God's microtape – which presumably contains the secret of the curability of
her lung cancer – is the object of the patient's apparently upbeat optimism. The
attending physician recognizes this as follows:

 1 MD: Which is fine. (1.0) Nobody wants to (0.2) encourage you ↑not to
 2   be optimistic. (0.5) The question is: (0.5) well- (.) may I <u>ask</u> a direct
 3   question? (0.8) What's going ↑on with <u>you</u> and what does it mean. (0.4)
 4   What are the main (0.2) <u>medical</u> problems you're con↑fronting right
 5   now. (1.8)
 6 Pt: The brea↓thing. (0.5)
 7 MD: Okay. (0.8) And what's the ↑matter with ↓it. (0.5)
 8 Pt: I can't ↓breathe.
 9 MD: Okay. (1.0) And do you know why <u>that</u> is? (1.8)
10 Pt: >Because I got ↑tumors.<
11 MD: Okay. (1.2) And (0.5) what are the <u>treatments</u> for those tumors? (1.0)
12 Pt: There isn't any.=But there could <u>al:</u>ways be a <u>magical</u> thing.=I be↓lieve.
13   (0.8)
14 Res: Gotcha. (0.5) Okay. (0.5) O↓kay.
15 Pt: I believe that <u>God</u> can °do <u>anything</u>,°
16 MD: Okay. (0.8) So I want to see if I get you right. =You understand that (0.8)
17   your ↑breathing (1.0) is (.) in <u>peril</u>, (0.2)

18 Pt: Right, (0.8)
19 MD: >And that the <u>rea</u>son for the breathing being in peril< (0.5) is (.) the
20   ↑tumors (1.2) and there's no (.) no <u>hu</u>↑man (.) fixing of that. =There's
21   no treatment for that. (0.5)
22 Pt: Yeah.
23 MD: And you're ↑<u>hope</u>ful you'll get <u>better</u> nonethe↓less.
24 Pt: <u>Right</u>.
25 MD: >That's fair enough.< (1.5) <u>E</u>ven with the ↑hope I want to ask (0.8)
26   what do you understand will happen ↑if that <u>doesn't</u> happen. =If it
27   ↑can't be ↓fixed. (0.2) If God (0.5) doesn't (0.5)
28   [fix ↓that]
29 Pt: [To be ↑ho]nest with you >I'm not gonna look at it that way.> (1.5)
30 MD: Okay.
31 Pt: I know you might think I'm <u>weird</u> but- (0.5)

Through this intricate repartee, the attending Palliative Care physician and the patient are able to come to a working consensus that there are no human cures left for her to avail herself of, without God's express intervention, and that nonetheless survival and longevity is a reasonable objective in the theological framework she is committed to. In the following section, the physician confirms that he believes her assessment of the situation is normal, not "weird". When the attending physician gently hands the primary guidance of the conversation back to the medical resident, however, it is noteworthy that he, unlike the attending physician, is unwilling to grant the theocentric rationality that is guiding the patient's preferences. In line 3 below, the attending physician attempts to hand the reins of the talk back to the medical resident, but the family member seems to resist the pass-back in line 5.

1   MD: There's <u>nothing</u> weird about ↑it, =We want to talk about this in a way
2   you're <u>will</u>ing to and you want to. (1.2) The reason this matters though,
3   (.) >I mean I can pass to you<. =I don't want to steal. (0.2) I don't want to
4   steal. hh= You you have thoughts.
5   FM: >You ↑might as well< let him do all the talking. ((laughter))
6   Res: I'm ↑okay =That's okay, We can <u>both</u> ↑talk.
7   [It's working]
8   MD: [This man's] a very bright skillful <u>ta:lk</u>er too.=and I (.) >I can come in
9   the room and take over. =You know her better than I do.<↑Take it from
10   there where I'm go↓ing. (0.8)
11 Res: What's [con↑cern-]
12 MD: [I'm <u>not</u>] talking anymore.

13 Res: What's concerning us (0.2) you know I told you this morning I said (.)
14   I think it's important to be ↑optimis↑tic (0.5) but to remain ↑realis↓tic.

What we have seen here is the patient's success in conveying to the attending
physician a presentation of self that is considered irrational by some medical personnel, and which many cite as the cause of a pernicious trend toward prognostic
discordance. Yet the attending Palliative Care physician recognizes the elements
of her argument and acknowledges them openly, against the wishes of some of
her own family members. In lines 13–14, however, the medical resident in training
recasts this development as a desire to be "optimistic but realistic," a standard
phrase from end-of-life discourse that in fact contravenes the very premises of the
patient's position. The co-presence of these two physicians and their engagement
with this patient is illustrative both of the diversity of approaches in Palliative
Care, as well as of some emerging intergenerational differences in the techniques
older and younger generations of Palliative Care clinicians use to align with
patient self-presentations.

For **expressions of belief in God's curative intervention**, see 4.3. For
patients' **conscious decision to not think about negative outcomes**, see 7.4, 10.8,
6.4, 7.1, 10.8, 10.10. For **hand-offs between attending physicians and trainees**,
see 8.1, 2.3.

4.5 I'd grow pot

In this last conversation in this series on self-presentation and self-characterization
in Palliative Care consultations, we share a transcript of an interaction with a
patient using a speech-generating device due to the progression of a cancer of her
nervous system. The question we pose is:
1) How do patients who are using an assistive technology to speak achieve a
    holistic or meaningful presentation of self in Palliative Care settings? (on the
    phenomenon of turn-sharing, see Lerner 2002)

The patient in the following conversation self-identifies as a 66-year-old white
woman and as financially insecure, reporting Bachelor's-level education and
no religious affiliation. She has been diagnosed with a cancer of the peripheral
nervous system and spinal cord, which is advanced. She has "no idea" whether
she will live for a year, while her clinician-rated survival prognosis at the time
of the following consultation is three to six months. In fact, she lived more than
six months, i.e., longer than the follow-up window of this study. The patient
strongly ranks her end-of-life goals as "comfort over longevity," and she rates

her "global" quality-of-life over the previous two days at a six out of ten. The following portion of talk occurred during the first visit of the Palliative Care team. The clinician speaking is a Palliative Care physician fellow. Utterances that are quoted repetitions of the patient's speech through the assistive device are placed in quotation marks.

```
 1  Fel:   ↑One ↑thing I wonder about _____ um (0.4) if you::: (0.2) were to
 2         learn that your time were shor↓ter.=are there things that you would do
 3         ↑differently? (34.0)
 4  Sp:    ["No ↓work."]
 5  Fel:   ["No work?" ]
 6  FM:    "No work."
 7  Sp:    You had been working here be↑fore this? (5.8) ((laughter))(0.5)
 8         What did she ↑say?
 9  FM2:   She wants to grow ( ). ((laughter))
10  Pt:    N::o. (1.5) I'd grow pot. ((chuckle)) (3.8)
11  Fel:   It's a big job. (0.5)
12  Pt:    Yeah. (0.2)
13  Sp:    Mm-hmm.
14  Fel:   Yeah. (0.5) I won↑der um (0.8) would you think that, kind of (0.2) figuring
15         out what to do: with (0.5) the business that you're:: do↑ing:.=would that be
16         helpful for peace of mind no matter what happens? (12.0) Have people help
17         you. (1.2)
18  Pt:    Yeah.
```

Despite drastically constrained language resources, this hospitalized person is able to convey a captivating and clear characterization of her desires and imagination in the current circumstances. "I'd grow pot" is an assertion that, in its spare and unequivocal formulation, conjures a broad repertoire of cultural associations, ideas about lifestyle, place, political orientation, commercial and labor relations, etc. With the handful of patients in our study who use speech-generating devices, we find that they are often able to marshal more meaning and interactional impact with their contributions than many of those who speak without an assistive device, in part because they are prevented (by time and production constraints) from engaging in the kinds of euphemism and indirection that many longer-term patients are able to deploy with ease. Though it is beyond the scope of this study, we refer readers to the burgeoning literature on interactional speech pathology in Palliative Care settings for further inquiry (see Pollens 2012; Collins and Marková. 1999; Roe and Leslie 2010).

*For **patients using assistive devices to speak**, see 6.1. For **frankness and indirection**, see 2.1, 6.1–2, 7.3, 8.3, 8.5, 9.2, 10.12. For patients' **imaginings about how to best spend the remainder of their lives**, see 3.6, 10.12, 5.5.*

4.6 Insights and implications from Chapter 4

In these first three thematic chapters that make up Part One, we have divided into three chapters what are traditionally interwoven aspects of "getting to know each other" in the hospital setting: those of introducing the discipline of Palliative medicine, those of querying and speaking back to it, and presenting the (patient's) self against the background of the Palliative Care referral consultation. We recognize that these are not isolated types, and we do not assert that there is any particular regularity to them. They are indicative of this particular historical moment in broader socio-political discourses about death and health, health care and quality-of-life, identity in institutional contexts, and patient-centeredness vs. expertise and authority. Nonetheless, we do believe that the diversity of practices reflected here is indicative of how patients and families currently working through serious illnesses in hospital settings tend to inscribe themselves, critically or normatively, into institutional discourses. In Part Two of *Palliative Care Conversations,* we survey some prevalent modes of discourse that are salient throughout the conversations in our study, namely rapport-building, intralinguistic code-mixing, and speaking for others.

Part II: **Dynamics of the Interaction**

5 Irony and rapport

A perfectly tuned conversation is a vision of sanity [...] The satisfaction of having communicated successfully goes beyond the pleasure of being understood in the narrow sense. It is a ratification of one's place in the world and one's way of being human.

– Deborah Tannen (1981: 145)

According to Roget's 21st Century Thesaurus, *rapport* originates in mid-17th-century French usages connoting yield, bearing, intercourse, return, bringing-back. Rather than describing intimacy or trust *per se*, rapport is a diplomatic tool indicating a track-record of mutual benefit, which justifies certain features of intimacy, trust, and friendliness. It is thus not a good stand-in term for intimacy or trust, unless a demonstrated prehistory is in evidence by which *rapport* has been objectively earned. In medicine, for better or for worse, rapport – like its inscrutable kin-concept "bedside manner" – continues to be an ever-central vernacular descriptor of the social virtues of one or another physician (see Bigi 2011).

But in Palliative Care contexts, rapport is a different ideal than it is in health specialties where the common goal of curing disease is presumed. And, as we've explored in the first three chapters, patients and families tend to enter a Palliative Care consultation with most of their habitual presumptions about medical treatment intact, if not accentuated by constant interaction with other specialists throughout the day. From a Palliative Care perspective, confidence in one's physician or clinical team is not the same as confidence that they will pursue all avenues of curative treatment available to the patient and family. Rapport in specifically palliative settings is a still-evolving ideal, and the communicative and interactional textures of its development remain under-addressed in research.

Understanding rapport in Palliative Care requires a shift in the customary dynamics of hospital-based rapport expectations. Clinicians must develop a practical sense for how a patient's and family's desires may subtly differ from the traditional scripts of intervention and persistence prized in much hospital discourse. Often, the resources and tools needed to develop this sense include some that may seem out of place in the rest of the hospital. We begin with one such tool: dispensing with the niceties.

5.1 No you're not

In the following brief greeting, the Palliative Care clinician openly contradicts a family member already in the midst of phatic getting-to-know-you volleys, on the

https://doi.org/10.1515/9781501504570-005

basis that doing so may offer relief from the pressures of politeness. This exchange indicates how rapport functions somewhat differently in Palliative Care consultations than in other arenas of health care treatment, where optimistic investment in curative solutions is often rapport's most consistent interactional resource. Our questions in this short exchange are:

1. How do irony, disabusal, and divestment from conventional approaches to rapport often constitute the basis of rapport within Palliative Care settings?
2. When do patients and families find "dispensing with the niceties" to be a relief, as they seek to come to terms with the complicated questions that await?

The patient in the following conversation self-identifies as a 55-year-old white woman and as financially secure, reporting Associate's-level education and Christian religious affiliation. She has been diagnosed with a stage-four breast cancer. She believes she is "very likely" to live for a year, while her clinician-rated survival prognosis at the time of the following consultation is two weeks to three months. In fact, she lived five days beyond this consultation, i.e., drastically shorter than both her and clinicians' expectations. The patient strongly ranks her end-of-life goals as "comfort over longevity," and she rates her "global" quality-of-life over the previous two days – i.e., physical, emotional, social, spiritual, and financial quality – at a five out of ten. The following portion of talk occurred during the first visit of the Palliative Care team, and the clinician speaking is a Palliative Care nurse practitioner.

1 NP: How are you?
2 Pt: Fine.
3 NP: No you're not.
4 Pt: Oh, a <u>load</u>ed question. (0.8) ((laughter)) hhh
5 Sp: It's been a long hh well? no
6 Pt: No:, it's a po<u>lite</u> question, it's it's °a po↓lite ↓answer.°

Though we do return to this conversation in Chapter 9.1, here we highlight a brief moment in the beginning of the consultation that allows the clinician to earn rapport very early on in the exchange with a seriously-ill person she has just met. Not only does the clinician rebut the patient's reflexive response "fine" with a conventionally face-threatening contradiction "No you're not," but she follows this intervention up with the metapragmatic observation "It's a polite question, it's a polite answer." (On such low-grade assessments, see Lindström and Heinemann 2009.) This is remarkable for a first exchange between two strangers, as the clinician is willing to risk conventional rapport-building pathways by contradicting the family member's self-reported state of mind. In doing so, the nurse practitioner shifts the frame of rapport away from scripts of confidence, optimism, and putting-a-good-face-on-things and makes room for another symbolic order to unfold in which honesty outweighs optimism. In this choice, we see the nurse practitioner endeavoring to offer a kind of conversation that is a "vision of sanity," as Deborah Tannen (1981: 145) describes it, in a hospital context that has hitherto elicited from the family a potentially maddening array of optimistic stances. We note that in line 5 the patient's spouse begins to hedge with a story accounting for how things have actually been for them and why, but stops short, realizing that such accountability is not being requested. He then reverts to a simple "no," with which he aligns with the clinician's project of reorienting the conversation toward frank exchange.

For **metadiscursive and metapragmatic markers**, see 8.1, 9.2, 5.3. For **frankness and indirection**, see. 2.1, 4.5, 5.2–3, 6.1–2, 7.3, 8.3, 8.5, 9.2, 10.12.

5.2 Is that *Scrubs*?

Sometimes rapport never gets off the ground, and the elements that might have promoted it prove elusive to the clinician. In the following consultation, the clinician and patient trade taciturn observations about television shows, and their ability to communicate with one another through these observations is ultimately inadequate. We ask:

1) What kinds of cultural and media references can help promote rapport?
2) What does it sound like when a clinician does not have access to the repertoire or experience necessary to build rapport with a patient?
3) How do patients, clinicians, and family members knowingly or unknowingly use cultural and media references to create barriers to communication?

The patient in the following conversation self-identifies as a 63-year-old Black man and as financially insecure, reporting Bachelor's-level education and Christian religious affiliation. He has been diagnosed with a stage-four kidney cancer. He believes he is "very likely" to live for a year, while his clinician-rated survival prognosis at the time of the following consultation is two weeks to three months. In fact, he lived 135 days beyond this consultation, i.e., longer than clinically expected but much shorter than he himself expected. The patient strongly ranks his end-of-life goals as "comfort over longevity," and he rates his "global" quality-of-life over the previous two days – i.e., physical, emotional, social, spiritual, and financial quality – at a five out of ten. The following portion of talk occurred during the second visit of the Palliative Care team, and the clinician speaking is a Palliative Care nurse practitioner. The television in the room is on during the entirety of this consultation.

1 NP: When I came in, I saw that you were watching (.) <u>Scrubs</u> earlier?
2 FM: °Yeah.°
3 Pt: Scrubs? (1.2)
4 NP: >Have you ever seen Scrubs?<
5 Pt: Yeah. ↑No >I wasn't watching Scrubs?<
6 NP: Oh ↓yeah,=Are you a big Scrubs fan?
7 Pt: ↑No?
8 NP: No. (1.0)
9 Pt: No I wasn't watching s-s-↑Scrubs at ↑a:ll.
10 NP: Oh: okay. ((beeping)) I just saw it on ↓TV (1.5)
11　　May have only been on there for a short time.
12 Pt: Yeah. ((sound of plastic wrapper crinkling))

The television show *Scrubs* (2001–2010), playing on television in the patient's room earlier according to the clinician and the family member, appears to the clinician to be a good place to start a chat about how the patient has been doing. It depicts, he may presume, experiences that both he and the patient can relate to, without delving immediately into clinical matters directly pertinent to the patient currently. In line 9 above, after the patient's family member confirmed that *Scrubs* had been on, the patient emphatically denies watching the television show, but doesn't offer corrective information until the next exchange:

1 Pt: I was watching (.) um: (.) To↑day Show?
2 NP: Oh, ↑okay. ((static))
3 Pt: And then um: (.) Steve <u>Harvey's</u> right now. (2.5)
4 NP: °Mm-hmm.° (1.0)
5 FM: I thought you've seen that.
6 Pt: Steve Harvey is: ↑funny.
7 NP: Yeah. (1.8)
8 Pt: And those ↑guests he has, ↑so fun↓ny.(0.8)
9 NP: Yeah. (2.5)
10 Pt: Mm-hmm,
11 NP: Is that- yeah, that's (.) that's Jerry Seinfeld, ↑right?
12 Pt: Mm-hmm,
13 NP: Wo:w.=he's (1.2) he's looking older. (4.0)
14 Pt: Heh.

15 NP: So. =um, (2.5) uh- I know uh we talked about a lot yesterday.
16 Pt: <u>Mm</u>-hmm,

Typical of some Palliative Care consultations is the kind of exchange exhibited here, in which the nurse practitioner attempts to combine a form of social joining with a bid to establish common ground via cultural references. Intuitively, the television show *Scrubs* would serve well as a vehicle for discussing, if only obliquely, the realities and irrealities of hospital procedure, and as an opening for the clinician to gain insight into how the patient evaluates and relativizes his current experience of serious illness. The patient's contributions to the exchange above can be understood as competing with the physician's rapport-building project of attempting to establish common ground. "Steve Harvey is funny," is the patient's way of rationalizing his television-watching as not merely because "it was just on," like *Scrubs* was. But the patient utters the statement about Harvey's funniness in a stern tone that does not invite the clinician to share the common ground of humor, but rather to stake out an identity as someone who does things for a purpose.

The further implicature may then be that he intentionally did not and does not watch *Scrubs*, and therefore does not wish to reflect critically on the workings or experiences of hospital life, as experienced by a predominantly white fictional cast of characters. Rather, he wishes to watch, and by implication discuss, things that are pleasing to him, such as Steve Harvey and his "funny" guests. *Scrubs* is a fictional medical drama starring a majority white cast, while Steve Harvey is a comedian and moderator most preeminent in African American communities, having won for instance 14 NAACP Image Awards since rising from homelessness to stardom in the early 1990s. As they watch the television together, the clinician does not take up the patient's twice repeated "Steve Harvey" token. The clinician instead returns with a question about Jerry Seinfeld's surprisingly precipitous aging, a volley that highlights his own history of watching television shows with white lead actors and identifying with their biographical arcs. This exchange can thus be considered one of multiply cross-cultural pragmatic failure (white/Black, young/old, healthy/ill). The clinician's initial *Scrubs* volley meets with a counter-volley that he is not able to participate in. Unable and uninvited to open up for discussion the topic of Steve Harvey's humor, the clinician closes the rapport-building project and moves directly on to re-opening the topics of conversation they had discussed the previous day regarding goals-of-care.

For **cultural and media references**, see *5.3*. For **interactional saliency of race and ethnicity**, see *2.2, 5.3*. For **frankness and indirection**, see, *2.1, 4.5, 5.1, 5.3, 6.1–2, 7.3, 8.3, 8.5, 9.2, 10.12*.

5.3 That's the frustrating part right there

Some Palliative Care conversations are openly antagonistic, due in part to patients' justified frustrations about how infrastructural and informational deficits in communication between specialties negatively impact them. Clincians' patient-centered modes of speaking sometimes exacerbate such frustrations, because they once again prompt patients to perform as the center of responsibility for information management and portrayal. This leads to complaint sequences (Couper-Kuhlen 2012b; Dersley and Wootton 2000; Drew and Holt 1998a; Drew and Walker 2009) and open antagonism (Dersley and Wootton 2000; Heritage 2002; Heritage 2010; see also Goodwin 2006). In this conversation we also encounter features of lay diagnosis (Beach 2001; see also Sarangi 2001) derived from the patient's long-term involvement in hospital health care systems, customs, and language, compounded by his sense that the clinician is abdicating responsibility for information management. In this instance, we ask:

1) What pre-existing circumstances foment antagonism and discord in Palliative Care conversations?
2) What interactional features in Palliative Care conversations exacerbate pre-existing circumstances of antagonism?
3) What interactional features in Palliative Care conversations help to mitigate pre-existing circumstances of antagonism?

The patient in the following conversation self-identifies as a 45-year-old Black man and as financially insecure, reporting Associate's-level education and Christian religious affiliation. He has been diagnosed with a stage-four colon cancer. He has "no idea" whether he will live for a year, while his clinician-rated survival prognosis at the time of the following consultation is three to six months. In fact, he lived 79 days beyond this consultation, i.e., within the expected clinical prognosis. The patient is unsure whether he prefers comfort over longevity in the treatment of his illness, and he rates his "global" quality-of-life over the previous two days at an eight out of ten. The clinician speaking is a Palliative Care physician.

```
1  MD:  So I mean I just went through Dr. ____'s note when he first met you and-
2        and he had men̲t̲i̲o̲n̲e̲d̲ when he ↑talked to you that you were kind of a
3        straightforward ↑guy (0.5)°That you°(.) really liked people to be pretty-
4        (.) >pretty s̲t̲r̲a̲i̲g̲h̲t̲ with you and not waste your ↑time?< (0.5) Is that
5        accu↑rate? (0.5)
6  Pt:  ↓Yep. (0.5) 'cause you can't tell me how long you're gonna be (0.2) or
7        what we're gonna ↑talk about? (0.5) What ↑are we talking.
```

8 MD: >Because it completely depends on ↑what you have to say?< (0.5) ↑How
9   can I possibly know? (0.2)
10 Pt: <What will I have to say?> (1.8) All right.

The patient, having long become attuned to the discursive habitus of patient-centered clinical communication, appears uninterested in doing the symbolic labor of representing "his own perspective" for the clinician, especially after having been flattered with the attribution of straightforwardness. For her part, the physician is holding to the 'patient-centered' notion that hearing the state of things from his perspective is the *sine qua non* of a successful consultation. The patient then does, frustratedly, rehearse what it is that he understands about his current condition (below), but then promptly distances himself from that position. Being prompted to repeat back a litany of established clinical facts clearly irritates this person, giving him the impression that his capacities for expression are being used instrumentally and unduly for an undisclosed purpose. Corroborating this impression is the ever-present figure of the material medical "chart", where – he believes – the clinical facts of his case ought to be adequately enough housed to obviate such a recitation on his part.

1 MD: ↑So (2.2) ↑Can (.) I ((beep)) (1.2) can you tell me (0.5) ((beep)) what (.)
2   they- the other doctors have told you: about °what's going on with your
3   condi↓tion.° (0.5)
4 Pt: Oh my god. °Well I° ( ) (1.2) they said: that um (0.5) my (0.5) white
5   blood cell count is back up (1.0) I'm on a no li- no (.) no liquid nothing
6   di↓et.
7 MD: °Right.° (0.5)
8 Pt: I mean- I ↑know you got °all this information°.
9 MD: I- I know↑ but- (.) my
10   [interest-]
11 Pt: [That's the] ↑frustrating part right there.
12 MD: I know-
13 Pt: Because I ↑know you know these answers ↓already. (0.8)

Compounding traditional conceptions of asymmetry of power and knowledge in clinical consultations, this patient is inclined to call explicit attention to what he sees as disingenuity around who-knows-what. The physician, however, dissembles by pivoting to references to the medical chart alone:

1 MD: I know, (.) what (.) the chart says?
2 Pt: Okay.

3   MD: But I don't know (.) what (.) >how much of it you understand.< That's why
4   I'm ↓asking.
5   Pt: I- I understand ↑totally ((beep)) (1.0) I want ↑you to understa:nd.
6   MD: Okay (0.2) So help me under<u>stand</u>?
7   Pt: All right. =>What do you want to know?< ((machine beeps)) (1.8) Do you
8   want to know (0.8) ((machine beeps)) the: (0.5) ((machine beeps)) (0.8) ↑I
9   don't know where to begin with this. =My <u>stom</u>ach is not as (0.5) uh:
10   distended as before (0.8) Um: (1.5) ↑pretty much anything you <u>al</u>ready
11   know. ((machine beeps))
12 MD: °Okay.°
13 Pt: >I want to get bet<u>ter</u>, =I want to go <u>home</u>.= =I've been here for over a <u>week</u>?<
14 MD: Right. It's -
15 Pt: I came here four   [days after che↑mo:]
16 MD: [Sick of being here.]
17 Pt: ↑No it's >I want to be here so that I'm <u>monitored</u>< better in <u>here</u> than not
18   know what's going on when I'm <u>at</u> ↓home.
19 MD: ↑Right (0.5) Right ((machine beeps)) Are you having much <u>pain</u>? (0.5)
20 Pt: Not right ↓now.
21 MD: °↓Okay.° The pain medicine that you're on is hel<u>ping</u>?
22 Pt: It's ↓okay.

Here above, the symbolic responsibility of "understanding" is being tossed back
and forth, and the patient refuses to entertain the possible benefit of narrativizing
clinical information that is already contained in his medical chart. Both speakers
are repeating each other's words competitively – understand, get better, surgery,
option – but they continue to operate at cross-purposes with one another. The
clinician seeks tro elicit a vernacular, holistic narrative from the patient, while
the patient finds such elicitations to be an untoward burden.

1   MD: Do- do they <u>know</u> whether ↓you'll: (.) e- if this: (.) <u>block</u>age will ever
2   get better?
3   Pt: °I have no idea.° =They said they was ex<u>pec</u>ting it to get ↓better.
4   MD: Okay.
5   Pt: It hasn't gotten ↑worse?
6   MD: Right (0.5) So they're giving you the nut↑rition through the <u>IV</u>: in the
7   meantime: >because you haven't been able to eat< (.) right, (0.5)
8   Pt: °Right.° (0.8)
9   MD: Um (1.2) ↑so (.) I- I >what I hear from you is you're saying:< <u>obviously</u>
10   (.) >you want anything that we can think of that's gonna help you get
11   better you would- you would want to <u>do</u>.<↑right?

12 Pt: Right.
13 MD: Right. =What have they said about whether surgery is an option?
14 Pt: °Surgery is not necessary right now.°
15 MD: ↓Okay (0.5) °All right° (0.5) So they think that this place in the colon
16   that's blocked? is gonna get ↑better? (0.2) Like it's gonna: (.) shrink
17   or some↑thing? or? (0.5)
18 Pt: Pretty much.

This is a moment where the clinician is engaging in what we think of as over-vernacularization, somewhat common in many health provider speech genres including Palliative Care. The clinician is dropping her g's at the end of gerunds, while choosing to use non-clinical words like "shrink" with a kind of solicitous credulity. In the next instance, the clinician drops her pursuit of "big picture understanding" and decides to take the patient's statements at face value and align with them.

1   MD: °Okay.° All right. ((TV sounds)) (3.5) So is there ↑anything that we can do
2   to help you with: your: com↑fort to help you get through this hospitalization:
3   (.) °anything.° (2.5)
4   Pt: As far as what.=pain?
5   MD: Anything. (2.5)
6   Pt: That I can think of? =What ↑can you do?
7   MD: >Minimize the number of people who come and ask you all the same
8   questions?<
9   Pt: That they already know the ↑answer to. =That's the killer part. I'm- I want
10   to bet the house you knew you al::ready know the answers to everything
11   you just asked ↓me. (0.2) >You know that's my breakfast lunch and dinner
12   ↓right there.<
13 MD: Yeah.
14 Pt: You know I can't drink.
15 MD: Yeah.
16 Pt: I can't eat. =Did you know that? (0.5) You knew that right?
17 MD: I- I knew: that they were not wanting you to =I didn't know whether you had
18   tried and whether you had gotten sick and how that experience was for you.
19   I'm trying to understand things from your perspective. (1.0) That's the
20   whole thing is. That's my job: to understand things from the ↑patient's
21   side and not be so focused on all the little numbers and details. =So
22   I'm interested in- how we can help your quality of life. That's my job.
23   [...] I don't know you and I haven't met you before and so I'm trying to
24   understand things from your side.

25 Pt: Well ↑↑ not a whole lot to say from my side, I'm in the bed? There's no cure (1.5).
26   They just want to shrink it, I'm pretty sure you're familiar with stage four
27   colon cancer, OK, so, can that be fixed? Or just shrunk. What's <u>your</u>
28   experience. And your knowledge.

Here is another instance where the clinician tries to over-vernacularize, by calling clinical data "little numbers." The patient responds by taking the clinician's self-negation at face value. It is noteworthy that he never throughout the conversation acknowledges she is a physician. By saying "I'm pretty sure you're familiar with stage-four colon cancer," a volley that would generally belong to "doctor-initiated talk," he essentially reverses their symbolic roles.

1 MD: It d-depends on what's already been done there,= And I honestly don't know
2   the answer to the question of whether this mass in your colon can be shrunk
3   in some way,= Or whether this is kinda there to stay. [...] I'm not really sure
4   what the p- how much better it's gonna get.
5 Pt: Neither am I, ma'am. That would be an awesome question for you to ask
6 MD: That would be helpful for you to know
7 Pt: Well, for YOU.
8 MD: Right
9 Pt: To ask the doctors.

Noteworthy here is that the physician self-corrects, just as she is about to use the word "prognosis," replacing with a vernacular "how much better it's gonna get." At one point in the conversation the clinician explains what Palliative medicine does:

1 MD: So we're sorta experts in pain management, and also in decision making,
2   so part of part of why I was here is–
3 Pt: You mean life-expectancy type decisions?
4 MD: Um ↑yeah, but ↑mostly to understand where you're, making sure you're
5   getting all the information that YOU need to understand what's going
6   ff-forward and to make decisions for yourself. So I don't have an agenda or
7   anything, I just wanna make sure you.
8 Pt: I didn't feel like you had an agenda.

Here again, the patient is enunciating concepts like "life expectancy" that historically have belonged to hospitalese, but now take the clinician off-guard because of their frankness. The patient's positive face threat above reveals the tension around Palliative Care's self-definition in this particular situation, but also in contemporary political landscapes. The clinician's response to the FTA is to acknowledge the potential perception that she has an "agenda", namely, to convince the patient to pursue comfort-only care. This leads to the following confrontation.

1 MD: You're a hard (0.5) you're hard on me! ((Laughter))
2 Pt: No I'm not, no I'm not! I'm the one in the bed.
3 MD: I know. I'm trying to underSTAND!
4 Pt: Well, I hope you're getting it? Cuz if you're not, the recorder is.

Here the patient recruits into his interpretive frame the audio-recording device used to record the conversation, harnessing the institutional symbolic power of objective research to buttress his own stance. At this point the clinician tries to recast the conversation and to recapitulate its take-away message.

1 MD: Can I summarize that your goal is to get better enough to get more
2   chemotherapy and hopefully keep this thing at bay.
3 Pt: That is the goal. Because I didn't sign up for C-diff.
4 MD: Yeah. It's no fun.
5 Pt: So _na_turally, quite _na_turally, the OBVIOUS is that I want to get back
6   to chemo so that. I'm not even in the _fight_ if I'm not getting chemo, right?
7   That's the obvious.
8 MD: Right.
9 Pt: That's the frustrating part right there, cause <u>Stevie</u> Wonder could see that.

It would be tempting to agree with the patient, that even "Stevie Wonder could see" that "I want to get back to chemo," and that the problem driving this conversational exchange in the direction it has taken lies simply with a physician's disingenuous inability to perceive the obvious. This assessment however forgoes the opportunity to track the intricate ways in which both speakers are symbolically inhabiting the position they assume to be of most value to the other: the patient speaking like what she imagines a physician speaks like, and the physician speaking like what she imagines a patient speaks like. Such mutual discourse prospecting does not arise in a vacuum, nor is it simply a result of symbolic role reversals. Patients, family members, researchers, and clinicians are position-takers in a complex political economy at work that was unimaginable only 25 years prior. The institutional savvy of the patient collides with the clinical habitus (of the physician) that tends to rhetorically disown its presumptive stance as bearer-of-knowledge. Meanwhile the politicization of end-of-life medicine has meant that physicians have been trained to avoid terminology like "life-expectancy" and "end-of-life," even as they guide the Palliative Care treatment.

For **cultural and media references**, see 5.2. For **interactional saliency of race and ethnicity**, see 5.2, 2.2. For **frankness and indirection**, see 2.1, 4.5, 5.1–2, 6.1–2, 7.3, 8.3, 8.5, 9.2, 10.12. For **lay expertise**, see 3.5, 8.1, 2.3, 10.7, 5.4.

5.4 Put them in the cornfield

In Palliative Care settings, rapport and irony are often mutually reinforcing interactional resources. In the following conversation, dark humor about institutional norms and procedure assists the family and clinician to establish a kind of intragroup trust (Gramling and Gramling 2012). The question we pose here is:
1) How do conversations that draw on irony and dark humor help establish a collective epistemic stance through which patients and clinicians co-construct their deliberations?

The patient in the following conversation self-identifies as a 77-year-old white man and as financially secure, reporting Bachelor's-level education and no religious affiliation. He has been diagnosed with an advanced cancer and has suffered a massive intracranial bleed. His spouse believes his prognosis is "poor", while his clinician-rated survival prognosis at the time of the following consultation is fewer than two weeks. In fact, he lived 3 days beyond this consultation, i.e., concordant with both family and clinical expectations. The clinician speaking in this conversation is a fourth-year medical student, and is joined later by a Palliative Care physician.

	Dt:	Can we ask you ↑questions?
1	MS:	↑Sure? If I can answer them I ↓can.
2	Dt:	Right. Well (.) I guess: Dr. ____ seemed kind of- I mean and him going
3		to this (.) ↑Palliative Care does that mean (0.5) about his: chance of
4		survival °are ↓slim to none?°
5	MS:	Yeah:.
6	Dt:	Okay.
7	MS:	↑Either =either =ei↓ther
8	Dt:	Well ↑he kind of answered.
9	MS:	Yeah: so,
10	Dt:	Okay. Now (1.2) if (0.5) there ↑is a chance he should get better which is
11		slim to none.
12	MS:	Mm-hmm.

13 Dt: Um: (.) then what <u>happens</u>?=Does he get to <u>stay</u> there? or: (.) does he: get

14   >kicked out as my mom said ↑booted out?< hhh

15 MS: Um:

16 Dt: hhh ((laughter)) What do they <u>do</u> with ↑them?=>Put them on the

17   ↑<u>side</u>walk?< hh ((laughter))

18 Sp: >Put them in the cornfield.< hh

19 Dt: >We're gonna yeah =>put him in the <u>corn</u>field?<He'd <u>go</u> >into the cornfield.<

20 MS: I think the <u>corn</u>field ahhh. =No: I mean =if- if- you know (1.0) very slim

21   chance that he ↓does-

22 Dt: Right.

23 MS: ↑Improve I- you know (0.2) whether he's going ↑home or a nursing home

24   I mean- (0.5) there's a <u>lot</u> of different <u>things</u> that (0.5) um (0.2) places that

25   you- you- you'd be. =wher↑ever's appropriate care-

26 Dt: Okay.

27 MS: For what<u>ev</u>er his <u>kind</u> of <u>functional</u> <status ↓is:.>

28 Dt: Okay.

29 MS: Uh it ↑won't be the <u>corn</u>field. ((collective laughter))

30 Dt: °It won't be the cornfield?° hh

31

The family in the midst of an initial Palliative Care consultation creates, spontaneously, a repertoire of laughter-worthy symbolic references – social tokens of in-group membership – which they then play off of the contributions of participating clinicians. Free of apparent malice or resentment, the family members nonetheless tactically reassert the primacy of their relationship with the patient, and – in so doing – gradually become unified in their support of a comfort-focused plan of medical treatment. Humor is the way they get to this resolution.

The family members, involved in a prognosis conversation, aggressively derail the official goals of the consult, and stage a coup d'état of sorts, reestablishing tentative control over the circumstances and the future, through recourse to a vernacular set of narratives about "the cornfield". Clinicians may worry that they have lost control of the consult, but exactly the opposite is the case. Taking the "long way around", the family goes through a series of social rituals that allow them to come to certainty about the next steps they will take. In the Palliative Care consult above, the official main focus of attention (Bolden 2006) is supposed to be a somewhat sober, situationally appropriate conversation between putative equals about the best possible outcomes for the patient. Nonetheless, the relatives seize the opportunity to disattend that main focus of attention, giving "the appearance of respectful involvement in their declared concern when, in fact, their central attention is elsewhere" (Goffman 1974: 201).

When the daughter says "put them out on the sidewalk", the thematic focus of talk seems to stay the same, but the rhetorical focus shifts markedly, as the family members begin to bait the unwitting medical student to either participate in, or exempt himself from, a string of talk that may be regarded as objectively offensive and therefore professionally precarious for someone like him who is – like the family members – relatively low in the hospital hierarchy. When the relatives issue an initial laughter token, and the medical student responds in kind, the relatives then "up the ante" by recasting the proximal, metonymic schema "sidewalk" with the distal, mythic schema "cornfield". They then wait to see if the medical student will return the bid. While the family members are purporting to talk about end-of-life planning, they are actually carrying out a much different intervention of their own, surveying the social landscape among clinicians to assess whom they will deem credibly unbeholden and authentic enough to joke – and joke well – about the death and dying of a beloved person. Such phenomena of patient-family talk, however, register rather awkwardly on the radar screen of Palliative Care best practices research, which has focused thus far on felicitous or infelicitous prognostic dispatch and uptake. This focus runs the risk of technologizing talk at the expense of examining the crucial social subtexts that make that talk necessary and possible. Cameron (2008) writes, "Talking to others ('communication') is an area of modern life in which expert systems are asserting themselves over more traditional, informal, and diffuse ways of organizing knowledge and practice. Discourse is being 'technologized', acquiring in the process its own specialist technologists – researchers, designers, and trainers." Clearly, the family's recourse to "the cornfield" signaled an insistence on the value of vernacular spaces of communication on one's own terms – of making true, meaningful sense of the world in a moment in which the illusion of technical omnipotence has been revoked for them.

The medical student was not left alone in the room for long. When the attending physician returns from an errand, he poses the reverent, honorific question:

1 MD: He was an active (0.5) man?
2 FM1: Yes he was. Very.
3 MD: Engaged in the world, Expressed wishes, about what he would want
4 should something like this happen,
5 FM2: Yeah, go in the cornfield.
6 FM1: This is a- (0.5) an inhouse joke. You put him out on the rocks.
7 FM2 He was a very simple person. ya know? Nothing fancy about him.
8 I don't mean simple.
9 MD: Leave him out for the wild animals? Well it's against hospital regulations
10 (.) we'll just leave him at the mercy of doctors.
11 ((Relatives laughing))

12 MD: Well I think part of our job is to protect him against doing things that would
13   make him more uncomfortable.
14 FM1: Right.
15 MD: And and so, all kidding aside that often is a struggle because um, we
16   always ask ourselves should we be doing something more something
17   different, and if it seems that that is the case we would talk to you about
18   it. At this point, focusing on comfort seems to make a lot of sense. Are you
19   all in agreement about this?

Now assembled as a united front, the relatives, together with the medical student, have established a shared symbolic vocabulary – to which the attending physician was not yet privy. Yet since they had already tested the limits of the appropriate misuse of humor with the medical student, the relatives feel on stable enough footing to spoil the intrigue and reveal to the physician that "this is an inside joke," thereby generously issuing to him a free offer of membership in their speech community. It is also important to notice that the physician's confirmatory volley around comfort-based care comes immediately after he is consecrated as a member of the "cornfield club" (see Egbert 2004).

For idioms of **leisure and the outdoors**, see 3.1, 4.1. For **expressions about going home**, see 4.1, 10.12, 4.5. For further examples of **social joining**, see 2.1, 3.1. For patients' strategies for **status recognition**, see 3.5, 8.1, 5.3, 2.3, 10.7. For instances of discord between **frankness and indirection**, see 2.1, 4.5, 5.1–3, 6.1–2, 7.3, 8.3, 8.5, 9.2, 10.12.

5.5 He's had this amazing ride

Rapport continues to be an important interactional quality in Palliative Care consultations up until, and beyond, the death of a patient (Roe and Leslie 2010; Abbot et al. 2001). In the following conversation, members of the clinical Palliative Care team are discussing with family members the logistics of withdrawing life support from their loved one. They discuss what the signs and thresholds of dying will be and then reflect on the patient's overall experience. We note in this conversation that irony and dark humor play an important role. The questions we ask are:

1) What do expressions of affiliation, rapport, and solidarity look like at the end of a course of Palliative Care treatment?

2) What sorts of resources and rituals are invoked to honor the patient as an active participant in his/her treatment and as an autonomous being, independent of his/her illness?

The patient in the following conversation self-identifies as an 82-year-old white man and as financially secure, reporting Bachelor's-level education and Christian religious affiliation. He has been diagnosed with a stage-four kidney cancer. His spouse believes he is "very unlikely" to live for a year, while his clinician-rated survival prognosis at the time of the following consultation is 24 hours. In fact, he lived one day beyond this consultation, i.e., concordant with family and clinical expectations. The patient's spouse strongly ranks their end-of-life goals as "comfort over longevity", and rates the patient's "global" quality-of-life over the previous two days at a zero out of ten. The clinicians speaking are a Palliative Care physician and a Palliative Care nurse practitioner.

```
1  MD:  But it could g- it could go right immediately or it could be you know-
2  NP:  [↑Minutes]
3  MD:  [Minutes ] to an hour or two something like that (0.5) It's some =it's some
4        (0.8) you know just so you're (0.2) are aw- are aware
5        [that might happen]
6  Dt:   [And Dr. ( )___] >his medications available ↑right at the ready?< So if he
7        were to show [any sign of distress. ]
8  NP:              [Of distress no.      ]
9  MD:   [He's not gonna ] °he's not gonna sit there. =No he won't.°
10 NP:   ( ) sit there in distress.
11 Sp:   He's actually (1.0)
12 SiL:  Yeah. (0.8)
13 Sp:   So. (0.2)
14 MD:   Yeah and we'll we'll give him before we unplug him a (0.2) good bolus a
15       little bit more °than what we've giving him as well.° (3.0) But he's had-
16       he's had this a↑mazing ride.
17 Sp:   That's good.
18 MD:   I mean ↑how long how long has this thing been?
19 Sp:   [He's had this a little over six years.]
20 Dt:   [Six years.                          ]
21 MD:   [Six years.                          ]
22       That's what I that's what I had thought. =I mean that's:: (0.2) ↑that's (.)
23       a ↑good ride. =Yeah that's a lot longer than-
24 Dt:   He's ↑done so well.
25 MD:   Yeah I ↑know he ↑has (.) Despite despite l-little thises and ↑thats and
26       then (.) and in fact he's not dying from ↑that.
27 Sp:   ↑No. =↑No
28       [((laughter))                        ]
```

29 MD: [He's dying from the ↓cancer] really which makes everybody <u>here</u> feel
30   ↑really good.
31 Sp: <u>Yes</u>:: <u>yes</u>: hhh ((laughter))
32 MD: hh

In line 18 above, the talk shifts from the "logistics of dying" theme to a broader view on the patient's years-long course of treatment for complications related to his kidney cancer. There are a number of metaphors in lines 14–16 that may sound coarse or ill-conceived, including the expression "unplug him" and the idea that his end-of-life experiences have been tantamount to "this amazing ride." But what becomes clear here and later in line 12 below is that the physician is speaking in such a way as to recognize the patient's spouse as a ratified participant in the "back-stage" talk of the hospital (Barton 2004) – the phrases, metaphors, and conceptions that tend to be used only among physicians and nurses in inter- and intragroup communication in the absence of listening or overhearing patients. This is not a case of disregard for pragmatics or the nuances of speech genre and audience design, so much as it is an intuitive stance (on the part of the physician) to regard the spouse and the patient as insiders in the business of health care – as veterans, rather than civilians.

This is a dynamic, we suspect, that is somewhat specific to Palliative Care relationships, where ambivalence about the norms and protocols of hospital life render health care as something to be experienced reflectively as much as it is to be consumed aggressively. The physician's disclosure about the patient in line 29–30 above, that "he's dying from the cancer really, which makes everybody here feel really good," is particularly interesting in this regard.

1   Dt: ↑That will (0.8) You <u>did</u> everything. =Yeah.
2   Sp: ↑Oh I'm -
3   Dt: He did ↑everything.
4   SiL: To the ↑T.
5   Dt: =Did it all.
6   MD: Yeah.
7   Dt: It can really sort of give me a ↑smile thinking about him.
8   FM: I know it.
9   Dt: [Amazing.]
10 FM: [Me too.] ((laughter))
11 Sp: [Yeah well.]
12 MD: Well he was a ↑<u>poster</u> child for the Palliative Care Group we put him ↑on
13   our uh
14   [our uh annual   ]
15 NP: [Oh he is on our brochure.]

16   I ↑saw him.

17 Dt: He ↑is on your <u>bro</u>chure. =He said that.

18 Sp: He ↑is on your bro<u>chure</u>?

19 MD: Yeah.

20 NP: He could be on the brochure ( ). Cool?

21 FM: Yeah.

22 MD: ((chuckles)) (1.2)

23 NP: For ↑Palliative Care when you want to ↑live. (0.2)

24 MD: Right.

25 SiL: That's right.

26 Dt: It's ↑true.

27 FM: ↑Yeah.

28 MD: ↑Right right.

29 NP: >How to get (.) get a <u>bet</u>ter life.<

30 Sp: <Tha:t's true.> True.

31 MD: So ↑are there o↑ther: <u>fam</u>ily <u>mem</u>bers: who- yeah.

This is a profound set of exchanges not only because, while the patient is actively dying, the Palliative Care physician is discussing how the patient will appear on the brochure for the Palliative Care service as someone who figured out "how to get a better life" amid serious, life-limiting illness. In that respect, the physician is continuing the intuitive, performative project of recognizing the family as experts and models in the endeavor of Palliative Care rather than as consumers of it. The discussion participates in the discourse of graduation rituals, where the successful graduate is praised by faculty as their 'pride and joy'. Furthermore, however, the physician, spouse, and nurse are also collaborating in the ongoing production of new ways to present and represent Palliative Care (see Chapter Two), thinking out loud about new brochure slogans and taglines. All of this could be construed as inappropriate for the context of a patient's active dying process, but instead we believe it is a complex form of recognition and ratification of lay experts (patients and families) in an overall vision to reform the discourse of health care in the United States.

For **metaphors of dying**, see 3.2, 10.1, 4.3, 8.4. 3.6. For reflections on the **patient's health history generally**, see Chapter 9. For **back-of-the-house talk shared with patients**, see 7.6, 7.4, 5.1, 7.2.

5.6 Insights and implications from Chapter 5

Though rapport is a desirable feature and outcome of all health care conversations, it manifests in surprising ways in Palliative Care settings. Often featuring jokes at the expense of the hospital and its customary procedures, rapport-building sometimes requires clinicians to deftly reorient themselves to traditional modes of expertise and authority and to the customary speech genres of neutrality and optimism. Some patients referred for Palliative Care consultations have a necessary investment in resisting rapport-building endeavors on the part of clinicians, especially if they disagree implicitly with their oncologist's decision to make a Palliative Care referral in the first place. But in some cases, the potential for rapport is scuttled by conflicts around culture and identity, or by misgivings patients may hold regarding the linguistic practices of patient-centered medicine, which they view as burdensome or euphemistic. In Chapter Five we have endeavored to represent a spectrum of such cases, which account for the specificity of this particularly nuanced context of health care communication.

6 Codemixing, multimodality, and speech genre

Though participation in this study required patients or their surrogates to be able to speak English, this methodological monolingualism – a significant limitation of the study – does not prevent us from learning from *intra*lingual speech diversity. This may take the form of stylistic and lexical variation in the ways participants in conversation design their contributions and the way assistive technologies (like speech-generating devices) create variation in the styles and interactional syntax by which participants communicate. Serious illness also tends to engender a kind of intrasubjective codemixing, in that hospitalized persons are often unable to engage in the full range of expression they would expect of themselves without illness, and this constraint brings forth in their contributions novel forms of making-do with the language they can command in the moment. It is in this nuanced sense that we turn to phenomena of codemixing and "translanguaging", a term applied linguists have been using in recent years to understand the ways people use their "idiolect or linguistic repertoire without regard for socially and politically defined language labels or boundaries – in order to make sense, solve problems, articulate one's thought, and gain knowledge" (Li Wei 2016: 4).

But codemixing, in the way we approach this concept, may also include complex forms of interdiscursivity (Park 2017), where participants may be layering various historical discourses about death, illness, and dying upon one another unevenly in the course of a given conversation. One participant may be evoking "mercy killing" or "euthanasia", (Dowbiggin 2003; Hyde and Rufo 2011), which are indices of political discourses that have been used to controversialize end-of-life care and Palliative Care in the United States since the 1990s. Often, these discourses are invoked preemptively at the political level in contemporary media discourse to rally citizens around a certain policy cause, and patients sometimes bring these anachronistic or politicized usages into their current interactions with hospital-based clinicians. "Anachronistic" may not be quite the right word, because we wish to be careful not to assume that the current institutional framework of Palliative Care is more morally, politically, or existentially germane than previous discourses on death. But this chapter nonetheless calls attention to the ways in which a heteroglot (spatial, temporal, cultural, and institutional) diversity of discourses and resources attends each of these consultations. Such phenomena have already been prevalent in the previous chapters, but Chapter Six focuses on them explicitly.

https://doi.org/10.1515/9781501504570-006

6.1 Do I have a future?

Consultations with patients using voice-assistive technologies, such as the following, bring forth phenomena of code-mixing and stylistic non-alignment, due in part to the effort and time it takes patients to produce the message and for family or clinicians to interpret and paraphrase, if necessary. But what these assistive technologies bring forth for our apprehension is a compromised patient's stripped-down, truncated repertoire of interactional resources, which are nonetheless able to contribute to communication in a differently meaningful way. In our presentation of this conversation, we ask:

1. What interactional features emerge in part by virtue of the stylistic constraint of the speech-generating device?
2. What unique stylistic power inheres in these mediated contributions, which may not be able to come forth in other forms of unconstrained speech in interaction?

This patient self-identifies as a 63-year-old woman and as financially insecure, reporting Bachelor's-level education and no religious affiliation. She has been diagnosed with a rare neurological tumor, the staging of which is not known or clear. She believes she is unable to estimate her prognosis, while her clinician-rated survival prognosis at the time of the following consultation is two weeks to three months. In fact, she lived more than six months after this conversation, i.e., beyond the follow-up period for the research study and therefore significantly beyond clinical expectations at the time. The patient strongly ranks her end-of-life goals as "comfort over longevity," and she rates her "global" quality-of-life over the previous two days – i.e., physical, emotional, social, spiritual, and financial quality – at a six out of ten. The following portion of talk occurred during the first visit of the Palliative Care team. The patient in this conversation is communicating using a voice interpretation device. The clinicians speaking are a Palliative Care physician fellow and a Palliative Care nurse practitioner. The long pause in line 4 below accounts for the time during which the patient was using the assistive device to formulate a response, and she communicates non-verbally between line 16 and 17, prompting the nurse practitioner's emphatic response in line 17.

1 Fel: The <u>last</u> time you didn't want radia↓tion, and you were worried about
2   having the ↑trach and the- the ↑PEG fore↓ver: (2.5) Now that we're ↓back
3   in a similar situa↓tion: (2.2) I think it's important that we, (.) find out what
4   your ↑hopes for the ↓futur:e are: (34.0) ((sound of an alarm))
5 Pt: <Do I <u>have</u> a future?> (2.5)
6 Fel: I <u>think</u> (1.2) there are still some <u>choices</u> to be ↓made:. (9.0)

7   MD: [So].
8   NP: [↑It's so hard] for any of us to know how much tim:e is ahead of us =>Is
9   ahead of ↑you< It's hard for us to <u>know</u> that at this moment=>There are
10   some pieces of information:< (.) that I think would still be <u>helpful</u> to have
11   that (0.8) understanding. (3.5) Is <u>that</u> something you want to know ↑more
12   about? (1.5) >it's kind of what other people who have been in a similar
13   situation< have experienced? (2.8) Nobody's had this: =It's a ↑<u>really</u> rare
14   type of tumor.=>But if <u>that</u>'s a piece of information< that's important to
15   you, we can help you get that information. (4.0) ↑Yeah (0.8) okay (1.5)
16 FM: Just kind of shoo↓ting in the dark, huh?=Yeah.=↓Yeah. (12.0)
17 NP: ↑Wow =Wow =↑Yeah =↑We're <u>all</u> feeling that way, too, and we're <u>so</u>
18   sorry for this news. (6.0)

This conversation challenges the limits of our methods of transcription, because we are unable (using the audio recordings sanctioned by our study protocol) to ascertain what the patient is saying or indicating in lines 16 onward. These are clearly turns at talk in which the patient is meaningfully participating, but we are only privy to the interpretations of the patient's words that are provided by the nurse practitioner in lines 12–13 and by the family member in line 16. But what is striking to us is the multimodal and intersemiotic nature of this communication. From the point of conversational conventionality, it is an extraordinary feature in line 5 that a full 34 seconds pass as the patient articulates a response to the Palliative Care physician fellow's volley in lines 1–4, in which he invites the patient to share her "hopes for the future."

Using her voice-production device, this patient returns the "future" token in line 5 above in a form that appears to be a rebuke, critically reformulating the hedge of the physician, and in a sense mixing up his code. The fellow's formulation in lines 3–4, "I think it's important that we find out what your hopes for the future are," appears to strike the patient as worthy of competitive recasting, as she undermines the physician's somewhat prolix "hopes for the future" volley with a bald, on-record question. Distinguishing between what the patient is able to say within the rhetorical restraints of the assistive technology and what she might have said otherwise would miss the point: that restriction enables different interactional resources – here, bold directness. The fellow's response, "I think there's still some choices to be made," deflects this directness, readopting the hedging jargon that was the object of the patient's implicit critique and explicit query. The patient and physician thus remain locked at stylistic and discursive cross-purposes. The patient, constrained by the resources of her speech-generating device and the time required to use it, issues an extraordinary, because unvarnished question that takes the clinicians off-guard.

It is worth noting here that this patient lived more than six months beyond this consultation, significantly more than was expected at the time. Thus the question "Do I have a future?" is no mere expression of desperation, but rather a substantive, informational query that, while outstripping the rhetorical resources the clinicians are providing in response, turns out to be a prognostically complex one. Nonetheless, the fellow's response that "there are still some choices to be made" in line 6 above is a faint and non-committal affiliation with the patient's query. The conversation continues with an equally unvarnished volley/query from the patient:

```
1  NP:   Yeah. (16.0)
2  Pt:   I would die here, (2.2)
3  NP:   Is that a question?=If- if you took the trach out would you::: die if we took
4         the trach out? =>Is that what you're wondering?< (1.8)
5  Fel:  Think that's what we're not (.) exactly sure a↓bout the, (0.5) And the
6         ENT doctors could tell us. (0.8) You know we can we can talk with them
7         more (0.2) after ↑this about (0.2) how (0.8) you know the reasons for the
8         trach and how much you really need it (.) and then we can report back.
9         (1.2) °And report what we learned from them.°=I know that (1.4) it's not
10        I know initially it was just for the bleeding but (0.3) it may be:: (0.2) you
11        know (0.2) like (.) the tumor might be kind of (.) °compromising the airway
12        also°.=°°So we'll have to check with them°° (3.5)
13 NP:   Yeah (.) these are all really good questions. (2.0) They're really (.) exactly
14        what you need to be (.) thinking: about at this moment. (3.5)  What to
15        expect (0.8) what to expect with the ↑trach (.) what to expect with the
16        tumor. (0.2) And I think there are- (.) I'm not just saying there's a couple
17        of people: (0.2) that we can bring in to that (0.2) ques↓tion. (0.8) Bring
18        into the (.) conversation.
```

The patient's summative conclusion in line 2, produced through the assistive technology, does not indicate prosody, intonation, or emotional cues that might allow the clinicians to appropriately align with her affective stance. In fact, it is not even clear from the machine-generated prosody if the patient is posing a question, or rather making a prediction based on the knowledge exchanged during previous several turns.

We understand this interaction as multimodal, cross-stylistic, and as code-mixing/translanguaging in nature, as the patient's contributions are what might normally be described as "curt", while the clinicians' responses and interpretations appear, in rhetorical context, prolix. Both patient and clinicians would appear here to be, under "normal" conversational conventions, flouting the Gricean maxim of Quantity and Manner (1975) – the clinicians with too much, and too prolix, information; the patient with too little and too blunt contribution. Yet these are precisely the affordances available in this interaction and are, as such, a helpful instance for appreciating the prosodic texture and sequential environment of any Palliative Care consultation that involves speech-pathological barriers or other constraints on the patient's ability to speak in a customarily fluent way.

For instances of **unexpected directness**, see 2.1. For **patients using assistive devices to speak**, see 4.5. For instances of discord between **frankness and indirection**, see 2.1, 4.5, 6.2, 7.3, 8.3, 8.5, 9.2, 10.12.

6.2 But isn't that like a mercy killing you know?

We noted in the previous conversation a circumstance in which the patient's ability to produce speech was curtailed, leading her to produce shorter and stylistically less indirect formulations. Such formulations are of course not always the result of physical constraints on the voice, and many Palliative Care patients interject such formulations into the consultation in ways that surprise their clinicians and clarify the moral, logistical, and legal stakes for patients and families. In this conversation, we ask how patients spontaneously endeavor to translate the contributions clinicians make into discourses that are familiar to them. At the core of this translative work are historical and civic discourses, often hotly debated in ages past, and in political, cultural, and religious contexts far afield of hospital medicine. What forms of such multi-layered interdiscursivity (Park 2017) attend these consultations, and what are their effects on the interaction?

The patient in the following conversation self-identifies as a 66-year-old white woman and as financially secure, reporting Associate's-level education and Christian religious affiliation. She has been diagnosed with stage-four lung cancer. She believes she will live for another year at least, while her clinician-rated survival prognosis at the time of the following consultation was two weeks to three months. In fact, she lived 11 days beyond this date, drastically shorter than her own expectations and somewhat shorter than clinicians expected. The patient is unsure whether she wishes to pursue care focused on comfort or longevity, and she rates her "global" quality-of-life over the previous two days – i.e., physical, emotional, social, spiritual, and financial quality – at a three out of ten. The following portion of talk occurred during the first visit of the Palliative Care team. The clinician speaking is a Palliative Care physician, working together with a medical resident training in Palliative Care.

```
1   MD:  >We want to be able to< help you ↑feel (.) as though (1.0) >this time is as
2        comfortable as it can be and we want to take away that worst symptom
3        which is< (0.6) ↑breathlessness for you. (1.5) And that (0.2) is >something
4        we have to be really ↑careful about:< because (0.5) you you are right,=we
5        can (1.0) >sort of step over that line to the point< where it would (0.2) it
6        would kill you? (0.8)↑Bu:t (.) the alternative- >you know there's gotta be
7        a medium ↑ground that we find,< and that's why we ↑have these
8        conversations >to be able to find< (0.5) how much do you want us to ↑help
9        you with that because (0.5) we have to find a middle ↑ground between but
10       [ we ↑can't let you be in that much,]
11  Pt:  [But isn't tha:t like    a mercy      ] killing you know?
12  MD:  It's ↑not mercy killing. (0.8)
13  Pt:  ((clears throat)) Now-
14  MD:  We're not doing it with the intention >of ending your life< at all.
```

Here the Palliative Care physician is describing how the clinical team would and would not seek to alleviate the patient's discomfort with breathing. Giving too much morphine, the clinician clarifies, might bring her "over that line" and "kill" her, and this is not what the team intends to do. Rather, in lines 7 and 9, the physician describes a "medium ground" of symptom-management that would allow her to remain comfortable, though her pre-consultation questionnaire indicates that she is unsure whether she wishes to prioritize comfort or longevity in her treatment decisions. In her query in line 11, the patient wishes to know if the procedure the clinician has described is "like" a mercy killing, indicating that she wishes not only to know not exactly whether such a treatment procedure "is" a mercy killing but also how "like" one it may be.

This is of course an appropriate, rational question for the patient to ask at this point in the interaction, and yet it catches the clinicians a bit by surprise, because it cites an older discourse about death and suffering that was hotly debated beginning in the 1920s and 1930s in the United States (Dowbiggin 2003; Hyde and Rufo 2001), and which remains a rhetorically powerful image by which patients and family members test the ethical and moral tenability of a prospective treatment decision. Euthanasia, mercy killing, and physician-assisted suicide are each complex historical discourses that structured the broader social imagination about death in clinical care in different eras prior to the ascendancy of Palliative Care in the United States around 2000. The discursive "code" around death that the patient is bringing forth is thus anathema to the vernacular the Palliative Care clinician will likely use in a consultation setting. And yet, the clinician has – in the course of his longer description of the comfort-measures approach in line 6 – suggested that under certain circumstances the treatment for difficulty breathing might indeed "kill you."

The physician does resolutely and promptly rebuff the "mercy killing" token in line 12 and proceeds in line 14 to address what has become the legal crux of palliative end-of-life treatment, which is the distinction between "hastening death" and "letting die." The decision in Vacco vs. Quill (1997) established this principle, based on the US Supreme Court's interpretation of the 14th Amendment as protecting a person's right to die, but not their right to be killed. Intention, then, is the crucial clinical, legal, and ethical yardstick which, as this clinician clearly indicates to the patient, translates into procedural decisions that "we have to be really careful about." In this brief exchange, then, we encounter a mix of discursive resources ranging from 1990s Supreme Court decisions to mid-20th-century moral and religious debates about merciful death (Dowbiggen 2003).

*For instances of **unexpected directness**, see 2.1. For instances of discord between **frankness and indirection**, see 2.1, 4.5, 6.1, 7.3, 8.3, 8.5, 9.2, 10.12. For exploration of **moral predicaments**, see 3.2, 4.4, 4.3, 6.2, 6.4.*

6.3 Did you have any spiritual or cultural beliefs?

In sharp contrast to the previous two conversations, which included surprising shifts in code and repertoire, participants in some Palliative Care consultations instead collaborate with one another to co-construct restrictions on which discourses or codes will be deemed viable in the setting. Patients and clinicians stake out mutually agreed upon regularities of discretion that they then observe together throughout the course of the talk. This is, then, not code-switching or translanguaging but rather code-management – i.e., the collaborative production of discursive boundaries. The questions that animate our observations in this conversation are thus:

1. How do patients and clinicians actively collaborate in producing internally acceptable ways of speaking (and not speaking) about certain topics?
2. How does this interactional production of discursive parameters differ, say, from merely designating proscribed or "taboo" topics?

The patient in the following conversation self-identifies as a 54-year-old white woman and as financially secure, reporting high-school-level education and Christian religious affiliation. She has been diagnosed with an advanced cancer of the Fallopian tube. She believes she is "very unlikely" to live for a year, while her clinician-rated survival prognosis at the time of the following consultation is more than six months. In fact, she lived 33 days beyond this consultation, i.e., shorter than clinical expectations. The patient strongly ranks her end-of-life goals as "comfort over longevity," and she rates her "global" quality-of-life over the previous two days at a seven out of ten. The following portion of talk occurred during the second visit of the Palliative Care team. The clinician speaking is a Palliative Care nurse practitioner. In line 3 below, we have omitted the name of the patient's prior place of employment, lest her anonymity be compromised.

1	Pt:	I worked <u>here</u>? (0.5)
2	NP:	You ↑did?. =↑Where'd you work? (0.5)
3	Pt:	_____
4	NP:	((laughter)) Well that's cool!
5	Pt:	Yeah.
6	NP:	So you ↑know some of these people huh?
7	Pt:	Yeah.
8	NP:	You have to keep them in <u>line</u> then. ((laughter))
9	Pt:	Yeah.
10	NP:	↑Okay. =Did you do you have any spiri↑tual or <u>cultu</u>↑ral beliefs that you
11		[↑wanna make sure] we're aware of? Okay
12	Pt:	[Uh::: no.　　]
13	NP:	Is there anything that helps you cope getting ↑through all this?=You've
14		<u>been</u> through quite a ↑bit over the last few years.
15	Pt:	[Yeah. Um.　　　　　　　]
16	NP:	[Been a busy ↑lady.] (0.5)
17	Pt:	No? (.)
18	NP:	No?
19	Pt:	'Cos the e:::: (0.2) It's been six ↓months well: it's been a <u>year:</u> and (0.8)
20		a (.) few months but um (0.8) ↑it's <u>been</u> six bouts of can↓cer. =↑That's
21		e↓nough. (0.2)
22	NP:	°Yeah yeah it's enough.° (0.5) You've ↑had <u>enough::</u>
23	Pt:	Yeah.
24	NP:	Yeah. =O↓kay. =Well there <u>is</u> clergy ↓here if you need.
25	Pt:	↑Okay.
26	NP:	If you want to speak to somebody (0.2) you know on a different- (0.8) you
27		know not a <u>medical</u> end but ↓just you know someone ↓to
28	Pt:	Yeah I-
29	NP:	That's ways available twenty-four ↑seven.
30	Pt:	Yeah.

30	NP:	So any↑time you just let us <u>know</u> or let the ↓staff know here. (1.0) Um (1.5)
31		↑so (0.4) it- it ↑sounds ↓like (0.2) um (0.5) one of the (.) things we would
32		need to do is just get a <u>prognosis</u> for you. (0.2) Um but it really sounds like
33		you're leaning more towards just being ↑comfortable-

In line 10, the nurse practitioner brings up "spiritual or cultural beliefs" as a kind of optional, need-to-know theme prompted by the clinical questionnaire, which is jointly dispreferred. "Spiritual or cultural beliefs" is isolated as an object that one has or does not have, and that one can disclose or not disclose. In framing her question in this way, the clinician draws an expeditious perimeter around this topic as an item that can be described summatively without opening it for exploration. In line 12, the patient responds with an equally preemptive formulation "Uh:::: no.", with which she performs *politely considering something undesirable*. The sequence from line 13–16 sees the clinician reformulate the question without explicit reference to "beliefs", but then in line 16 she inserts a positive stylization of the patient as a "busy lady", thus retracting the request that the patient disclose her coping techniques. "Busy lady" works as a laudatory attribution that projects logistical resilience and competence, requiring little or no help from therapeutic others.

The turn in lines 19–21 includes three tokens of "enough", in the sense of having reached peak reasonable tolerance – two from the clinician confirming the one from the patient (see Tarbi 2017). "Enough" in the patient's contribution appears to refer to her *efforts* in combating cancer, suggesting that she is not interested in further curative interventions. But the clinician's response "You've had enough" incorporates the previously introduced topical item of "spiritual and cultural beliefs" into her assertion, implicitly characterizing talking about "spiritual or cultural beliefs" as potentially *too much*. "Enough" is thus a mutual signal the clinician and patient trade with one another to indicate that they do not intend to talk substantively about "spiritual and cultural" beliefs. This kind of collaborative preemption of a topic considered potentially central to Palliative Care treatment and to end-of-life preparation is an instance of non-codeswitching, or the mutually agreed-upon willingness to leave an entire discourse or register of talk unbroached. It is included in this chapter in order to suggest that code-switching is not merely an additive phenomenon that occurs in a minority of interactional settings, but rather an ever-present and potentially transformative act performed collaboratively, between how one currently speaks given the discursive order and how one *might* speak when availing oneself of all the resources available under the transformative aegis of "translanguaging" (Li Wei 2016). In this conversation, the participants collaborate to narrow this range, rather than expand it, and they likely have good situational rationales for doing so, whether those be rapport-building, expediting treatment decisions, or alleviating anxiety.

*For instances of **proscribed topics**, see 2.3, 9.3, 3.3.*

6.4 I said "Doctor *I'm* the two percent"

Though all of the patients in the study are speakers of English, many speak English as a second or additional language. Here we present a conversation with a first-language Mandarin speaker who uses the ideological resources of US English in flexibly strategic ways. A question that motivates our exploration of this conversation is:

1. How do additional-language speakers of English harness the complex ideological resources of English, and particularly of US American English, to characterize themselves and their needs vis-à-vis health-care discourses?

The patient in the following conversation self-identifies as a 61-year-old Asian American woman and as financially insecure, reporting Graduate-level education and Christian religious affiliation. She has been diagnosed with a stage-four pancreatic cancer. She believes she is "very likely" to live for a year, while her clinician-rated survival prognosis at the time of the following consultation is two weeks to three months. In fact, she lived more than six months beyond this consultation, i.e., longer than clinically expected and concordant with the patient's own expectations. The patient considers her end-of-life goals as "comfort over longevity," and she rates her "global" quality-of-life over the previous two days at a one out of ten. The clinician speaking is a nurse practitioner student. In this portion of talk, the patient is reflecting comparatively on her own positive attitudes toward accessing treatment in hospital settings, as they contrast with those of another female advocate, whom she characterizes as easily "frustrated".

1	Pt:	↑She was (.) ↑frustrated right away. (0.6) I'm not frustrated. (0.3) I'm
2		straightforward. (0.4) Keep finding the ans<u>wer</u>.
3	NP:	Right. (0.5)
4	Pt:	You know how can I be helped? (0.2)
5	NP:	Right. (0.5)
6	Pt:	And I don't blame (0.5) their perfor↓mance. (0.5)
7	NP:	Right.
8	Pt:	That's not my job. =I'm just a ↑poor pa↓tient. (0.8) And ____ said (1.8)
9		Your problem (.) is going to end it <u>here</u>. (0.2) I'm going to go (0.2) and
10		tell the doc↓tor. (2.2) She was <u>frustra</u>↓ted (0.2) when she heard what
11		happened [to ↓me.]
12	NP:	[Yeah.] (0.8) Yeah <u>you've</u> been through a ↑lot. (2.2)
13	Pt:	<u>I</u> don't want to ↓die. (0.5)
14	NP:	No.

15 Pt: Don't want to die. (0.2) So the reason ↑I keep asking <u>quest</u>ion (0.2) I don't
16   want to die (0.6)
17 NP: And you seem like a very <u>very</u> strong woman. =So- (1.0)
18 Pt: I'm very [positive.   ]
19 NP: [You're doing every]thing.=↑yep
20 Pt: I'm very positive.
21 NP: I think that's the best medicine right there. (1.0) I can <u>tell</u>. (1.0)
22 Pt: (0.5) <u>you</u> have a tough cancer. (1.2) Survival rate is <u>only</u> (3.2) one ↓year (0.4)
23   the <u>most</u>. (1.2) And only two percent can make that. (0.2) I told him (0.8)
24   <u>straight</u> to his eyes (0.2) I said Doctor <u>I'm</u> the two per↓cent.
25 NP: Mm-hmm,
26 Pt: And he mentioned with post-surgery (0.2) the survival rate is one percent.
27   (1.5) I said <u>I'm</u> the one per↓cent.
28 NP: Yeah? (1.0) Good for you? (2.2) It's just a <u>num</u>ber you know. =You gotta
29   think about (.) your<u>self</u> and everything you can <u>do:</u>. (1.8) I know. (1.5)
30   Gotta keep your [head up.]
31 Pt: [I got to] fight.
32 NP: That's right.
33 Pt: The fight with cancer <u>che</u>mo (0.5) radiation.

Beginning in lines 1–2 above, the patient harnesses some of the more charismatic images ("straight-forward", "finding the answer" and in line 8 "poor patient") to characterize her compromised position in a health care institution that appears to have flagged in the ongoing pursuit of curative interventions for her stage-four pancreatic cancer. In this consultation, she is recruiting the Palliative Care nurse practitioner to her project of self-characterization as a statistically exceptional case. In lines 24 and 27, the patient appropriates the syntax of the circulating political discourse (around the time of this study) of Occupy Wall Street "We are the 99 percent" and refunctionalizes it for her project of modeling, for the nurse practitioner, her own performance of triumph over cancer. She does not say in response to the (absent) oncologist, "I will beat the statistics" or "I will be one of those 2% who survive," but rather makes a statement of *identity* in the present tense: "I am the (X)."

This is the epitome of creative translanguaging, in that speakers use and combine the idiolectal resources at their disposal to solve practical problems, regardless of which language, code, or culture these resources are attributable to. A further instance of translanguaging and code-switching ensues when, also in line 24 and 27, the patient switches from 2 percent to 1 percent in her persistent pursuit of affiliation and solidarity from the (absent) doctor. This flexible accommodation to the rhetorical imperatives of the moment, switching codes as necessary or prudent in the face of various forms of symbolic and institutional power, is an exemplary instance of communicative competence among so-called non-native speakers of English.

For examples of **optimism**, see 7.4, 4.4, 10.8, 7.1, 10.8, 10.10. For idioms and metaphors of **business negotiation**, see 10.3, 2.1.

6.5 Frankly my quality-of-life right now is not good

A final conversation in this chapter on codes and code-mixing concerns the ways in which patients attune to and appropriate a certain code in use among clinicians, producing critical insights from it that would not have arisen otherwise. In the following conversation, the figure of "quality-of-life" receives spontaneous and deeply productive scrutiny from the patient, who is unwilling to use it in the positivistic way that it has been presented to her in hospital discourse thus far. The question we ask therefore is:

1. How do patients "unlock" the codes of clinical discourse in ways that yield critical insight and practical benefit to them?

The patient in the following conversation self-identifies as a 72-year-old white woman and as financially secure, reporting Graduate-level education and no religious affiliation. She has been diagnosed with a stage-four ovarian cancer. She believes she is "likely" to live for a year, while her clinician-rated survival prognosis at the time of the following consultation is two weeks to three months. In fact, she lived 12 days beyond this consultation, i.e., shorter than clinically expected and much shorter than she herself expected. The patient is unsure whether her end-of-life goal is comfort or longevity, and she rates her "global" quality-of-life over the previous two days at a seven out of ten. The following portion of talk occurred during the second visit of the Palliative Care team. The clinician speaking is a Palliative Care nurse practitioner.

1 Pt: The i- (0.5) issue I've had in the last ↑week or <u>so</u> is that (.) I <u>mean</u> I
2   unders↑tand the idea that (1.0) you know (0.2) ((clears throat)) sometimes
3   (0.5) s↑topping treatment (0.2) the ide↓a of (1.5) uh (.) ((clears throat))
4   ((coughing)) (0.8) ↑you know (.) °it would give you a better quality° of ↑life
5   (.) but (.) very frankly my quality-of-life right now: is not <u>good</u>,
6 NP: °°Yeah.°° (0.5)
7 Pt: So I'm hhh it's like (0.5) uh hh (1.0) if I ↑knew that hh (1.0) that stopping
8   treatment would give me a better quality of ↑life for (0.5)
9 NP: Mm-hmm.

10　Pt:　Life for >a <u>shor</u>ter period of ↑time.<
11　NP:　Mm-hmm.
12　Pt:　I might ↑opt for that hh but that's sort of <u>like</u> the better quality of ↑life.
13　　　　(0.2) uh hh (0.5) as this- (0.5) it just <u>seems</u> like (0.5) <u>e</u>verything is going
14　　　　↓wrong. hh
15　NP:　°Mm-hmm. =Yes.° (1.0) You're [feeling]
16　Pt:　　　　　　　　　　　　　　　　 [And I'm] <u>not</u> on ↑treatment. (0.5)
17　NP:　°°Right. (.) Right.°° =And every day seems to be getting (.) °more
18　　　　uncomfor↓table.°
19　Pt:　↓Yeah.
20　NP:　°°Yes°° (0.5) So that is a- (.) that- that is our <u>high</u>est goal (0.5) is to (1.0)
21　　　　<start making you feel <u>better</u>≥ (0.2) by helping some of those <u>symp</u>toms
22　　　　°that are bothe↓ring you.° (1.0) <u>Absolutely.</u> (0.5) Um (0.2) because whether
23　　　　or not you get ↑treatment (.) ↑that should ↓be (0.5) ↑<u>high</u> prio↓rity.

Beginning in line 4, the patient deconstructs the term quality-of-life based on her observation that, since she is currently not on curative treatment regimens, a goals-of-care conversation predicated on the ideal of improving quality-of-life is illogical. This is a surprisingly infrequent feature of these consultations: that a patient calls into question the logic and semantics behind one of the primary tenets of end-of-life discourse without simultaneously resisting palliative approaches outright. We consider this an instance of code-mixing because the patient appropriates the charismatic institutional discourse and turns this element of the institutional code into an analytical resource of her own.

　　　For **critiques of quality-of-life discourse**, see 2.4, 3.5, 7.5 6.1–2, 2.1, 6.4, 7.3.

6.6 Insights and implications from Chapter 6

In this chapter we have presented five divergent instances of code-mixing, code-management, multimodality, and translanguaging, which demonstrate techniques patients and families use to manage interactional projects to their benefit. Certainly, future research will expand these conceptions to include conventionally understood multilingual and multidialectal data among speakers of languages beyond English in Palliative Care. Speech pathological and psychiatric insights into Palliative Care conversations are another area in which this research into code-mixing will continue to grow.

　　　Though English is the dominant language in evidence in these conversations, and English competency a precondition for patient participation, this is no reason to approach such consultations as monolingual or linguistically un-diverse.

Various speech genres, vernaculars, and sociolects are at work in complex constellations in these conversations, and they mark and position participants in meaningful ways. Seriously-ill speakers are facing physiological conditions for speaking and enunciating that alienate them from their conventional language habits, thus making "monolingualism" itself a practical impossibility, such that translanguaging becomes the norm and essence of their experiences.

7 Speaking for others

One of the primary and unexpected features of the Palliative Care conversations we studied is the way in which patients and family members strategically ventriloquate or mobilize the voices of clinicians who are not present. These may be oncologists, radiologists, other Palliative Care physicians, or the entire composite voice of the hospital setting, whether in the current moment, in recent interactions, or even in the distant past. This chapter is dedicated to understanding the complex function that these acts of "speaking for others" has in Palliative Care conversations specifically, and to revealing some of the ways that such acts of speaking-for impact the other primary themes of Palliative Care, including goals-of-care communication, symptom management, and end-of-life planning and discussions.

7.1 He basically didn't want to waste any more chemo on me

In the following conversation, a patient tries to communicate to a Palliative Care nurse practitioner his (absent) oncologist's stance about further curative measures, such as radiation and chemotherapy. Particularly, in this conversation, we are interested in understanding the nurse practitioner's persistent non-uptake of the patient's telling around the oncologist's stance. Our question is:

1. How do Palliative Care clinicians implicitly value the contributions of absent clinicians from other disciplines, when those clinicians' stances are portrayed by patients themselves?
2. What symbolic work gets done in interaction by invoking absent clinicians and through reported speech or summaries of those clinicians' stances?

The patient in the following conversation self-identifies as a 54-year-old white man and as financially secure, reporting Associate's-level education and Christian religious affiliation. He has been diagnosed with a stage-four colon cancer. He feels he is unable to estimate his prognosis, while his clinician-rated survival prognosis at the time of the following consultation is three to six months. In fact, he lived eight days beyond this consultation, i.e., drastically shorter than clinically expected. The patient strongly ranks his end-of-life goals as "comfort over longevity," and he rates his "global" quality-of-life over the previous two days – i.e., physical, emotional, social, spiritual, and financial quality – at an eight out of ten. The following portion of talk occurred during the first visit of the Palliative Care team, represented here by a PC nurse practitioner. The patient is summarizing for her the oncologist's current stance toward the treatability of his illness.

https://doi.org/10.1515/9781501504570-007

1 Pt: Um, he basically didn't want to waste any more (.) um chemo on
2   me, (0.8) because he said it was just not worth it. (0.5) But (.)
3   so did- (1.2)
4 NP: So Dr. _____ and Dr. _____ um (.) feel that the <u>chemo</u>therapy would ↑not
5   be bene<u>fic</u>ial but be more ↑risk?
6 Pt: ↑Well: I- I think Dr. _____ has a little bit of a (.) thought about it (.)
7   but (.) the other ones don't.
8 NP: Okay, ↑Dr. _____?
9 Pt: ↑Yeah, °Dr. ↓_____,° so.
10 NP: Right =And-
11 Pt: Because ↑I've, I've stumped them the last (.) <u>year</u>. (2.8) Every <u>time</u> they
12   give me radiation or- or che↑mo (.) I don't get sick? (0.8) There's no uh-
13   =like I said that's the worst thing I've had (0.8) My fingernails.
14 NP: Yeah.
15 Pt: I don't get ↑sick =I- I mean (.) the ↑first radiation I had I was getting sick
16   °off of it.°
17 NP: Okay.
18 Pt: Um, it wasn't <u>bad</u> but it w- I was getting a little ↓sick.
19 NP: Okay.
20 Pt: But uh they started giving me uh (.) some ↑shots. <u>So</u> that took away all the
21   uh (.) any, any nau↓sea.
22 NP: Okay. <u>Nau</u>sea. ↑Okay.

We are interested in how the patient here develops a scenario in which he has
"stumped" all clinicians' expectations, while the nurse practitioner engages in a
complex project, beginning in line 4–5, to interpretively recast the patient's report
in lines 1–3 as both reported speech and as tactical self-stylization at once. In
line 5, she recasts the oncologist's reported unwillingness to waste resources as
potentially a prudent weighing of benefits and risks to the patient, rather than as
an unwise expenditure. Palliative Care clinicians very often face predicaments in
how to treat patients' reports of other clinicians' stances. The nurse practitioner's
strategy in this conversation, in lines 4–10, is to individuate the various physicians
involved, so as to differentiate their various clinical recommendations, whereas
the patient is advancing a unified image of oncology/oncologists as having 'given
up' on him. The patient uses the polemical metaphor of "wasting" chemotherapy,
as one would speak of a precious commodity, and the nurse practitioner declines
uptake of this metaphor. Her non-uptake of the metaphor of "waste", together
with her attempt to individuate the various oncologists, who have been invoked
collectively, prompts the patient to pursue his project with a different set of fig-
urations, characterizing himself as a puzzle that has "stumped" the oncologists.

He is careful to fend off the nurse practitioner's concern about benefits vs. risks of chemotherapy by asserting that all potential side effects are minor (fingernail breakage) or easily cured (nausea). Through such moments of conversation, we are interested in how patients, family members, and clinicians themselves invoke the absent presence of another clinician who has been involved in the care of the patient.

For patient-initiated **metaphors of "the odds"**, see 7.5, 9.4, 4.3, 4.2, 4.1. For **patients' characterizations of curative treatments as a commodity**, see 2.1. For **attempts to interpret absent clinicians' stances**, see 2.2, 10.10, 2.3, 7.6, 9.5, 8.5, 7.5, 4.2, 7.2.

7.2 He's a lot better now at dealing with bad news

In some cases, patients' reported-speech characterizations of other, absent clinicians turn toward the language of empathy, care-taking, and tolerance. Strategic and informational motivations for reporting non-present clinicians' speech may persist, while simultaneously patients and families talk about what their primary care physician or oncologist has said or done, in order to show their admiration, empathy, or understanding of those clinicians' points of view as those of complicated human beings. The following conversation prompts us to ask:

1. How do patients tend to characterize and illustrate the complex humanity of other clinicians they work with?
2. How do Palliative Care clinicians respond to, or participate in, such characterizations?
3. What kind of symbolic work gets done through these joint characterizations of the complex humanity of absent clinicians?

The patient in the following conversation self-identifies as a 72-year-old white woman and as financially secure, reporting Graduate-level education and no religious affiliation. She has been diagnosed with a stage-four ovarian cancer. She believes she is "likely" to live for a year, while her clinician-rated survival prognosis at the time of the following consultation is two weeks to three months. In fact, she lived 12 days beyond this consultation, i.e., shorter than clinically expected. The patient is unsure whether her end-of-life goal is comfort or longevity, and she rates her "global" quality-of-life over the previous two days at a seven out of ten. The following portion of talk occurred during the second visit of the Palliative Care team. The clinician speaking is a Palliative Care nurse practitioner. The patient and her spouse are speaking about the oncologist's attitude toward further curative treatments.

1 Sp: °___ have you any uh- (1.0) <u>comments</u>°?
2 Pt: Nope not really. (7.5)
3 Sp: Did seem to get the idea that (0.5) going with this new thing (0.5) was (.)
4   what (.) ↑he would sug<u>gest</u>. (0.5)
5 NP: °That's okay. °
6 Sp: And we just <u>trust</u> him. (0.5)
7 NP: Absolutely. (1.2) Absolutely. (1.0)
8 Sp: >And <u>he</u> didn't seem to be <u>he</u>sitant< °about that.°(1.2) Again he (.) did ↑not
9   say that it had (0.3) ↑huge chances of ↑working. (1.2)
10 NP: °Mm-hmm.°
11 Sp: <u>But</u> (0.3) °he did say this was what he would do.°
12 NP: Um (1.8) and (0.5) and I would (1.0) <u>talking</u> about those same ↓things (1.5)
13   um (1.0) again (.) it's (.) it's: (0.5) part of the °( ) to come is° (0.5) because it
14   is really °°hard for him°° (0.6) But yet he <u>has</u> become so <u>fond</u> of you.
15 Pt: .hhhh I know he's a <u>lot</u> better now at uh (0.6) dealing with bad news than
16   he used to be. hh (0.5)

Here, what Erving Goffman would call the "official focus of attention" (1974) is
whether or not the patient should pursue a new curative therapy, the efficacy
of which is in doubt – both among the Palliative Care team and for the referring oncologist. The patient and particularly her spouse (in line 3) marshal the
oncologist's guarded skepticism about the treatment as a resource for justifying
pursuing it. His characterization of the oncologist as a rational, sober adviser
allows this absent clinician to enter into the interaction symbolically as a voice of
tempered reason, whose recommendations 'we' follow even in contexts of doubt.

But this official topic comes accompanied by another project, managed by the
spouse in line 6, 8, and 11, and by the patient primarily in line 15 above, of offload-
ing some of the empathic intensity of the current interaction onto the absent oncologist, who himself becomes a subject of the group's care, forbearance, and patient
nurturing. The absent oncologist's growth as a person and his ability to cope with
"bad news" overtakes, if only briefly, the centrality of the patient and family's
concern as the actionable locus for nurturance, growth, and change. The conversational "procedure" of Palliative Care has pivoted, thanks to the family's redirection
of it, toward their trusted though gruff oncologist. The intervention continues:

1 NP: You ↑know, (1.0) ↑that's (0.5) ↓that's (0.8) a great <u>compliment</u>. (0.2)
2 Pt: One time (1.0) uh- (1.2) I think it was my ↑first recur↓rence. (0.5) I went into
3   the office.=He told me what we were going to ↑do. (1.0) Uh (1.2) he ↓left
4   (0.5) and the (.) ↑nurse at that time was ( )
5 NP: Uh huh.

6 Pt: And uh (0.5) actually what happened was ↑he walked out of the room (0.5)
7   and uh (1.2) uh (.) he sort of looked to see if she was coming and (0.5) uh
8   she said 'Go ↑back to the office and do your paperwork' and talked to me.
9 NP: Ah ((laughter)). Yeah I can tell you some things.
10 Pt: Right.
11 NP: Yeah. Yeah.

The patient's unflattering story about the oncologist's prior aversion to conveying bad news is inflected as a telling about his redemption and growth. The Palliative Care nurse practitioner takes up this project, encouraging the patient's laudation of her oncologist by corroborating in line 9 the substantive grounds of the patient's compliment-paying. This collective face-work to benefit "difficult clinicians" and their emotions creates a cover for the patient to share negative experiences, and also for the nurse practitioner to share knowing intimations about the prevalence of such clinicians. In this way, the nurse practitioner and family form, or join, an epistemic community that shares a common, experientially informed stance toward the ingrained aversions to serious illness they have tolerated in hospital culture more broadly (see Atkinson 1995). Such may be considered one of the primary ways in which patients, families, and clinicians collectively socialize around the values of Palliative Care.

   For *patient-initiated* **characterizations of denial and/or empathy toward other clinicians**, see 7.5, 2.2, 10.10, 2.3, 7.6, 9.5, 8.5, 7.1, 4.2. For **clinicians' commiseration with patients' negative experiences in hospital**, see 7.6, 7.4, 5.1, 5.5.

7.3 I'm history

Beyond the informational, strategic, and empathetic invocation of non-present clinicians in Palliative Care conversations is a phenomenon we understand as an exegetical mode, in which patients take the clinical verbiage of an absent physician as a kind of text to be deciphered, and they translate it – sometimes quite confidently – into their own vernacular implications. Our questions are:

1. What kinds of interpretive practices do patients develop to discern the implicit stances of their clinicians of various specialties?
2. How might we characterize the overall literacy of discernment that patients develop through their multiple and continuous interactions with clinical personnel?

The patient in the following conversation self-identifies as a 78-year-old white man and as financially insecure, reporting high-school-level education and

Christian religious affiliation. He has been diagnosed with a stage-four kidney cancer. He believes he is "unlikely" to live for a year, while his clinician-rated survival prognosis at the time of the following consultation is three to six months. In fact, he lived 131 days beyond this consultation, i.e., concordant with his and the clinicians' expectations. The patient strongly ranks his end-of-life goals as "comfort over longevity," and he rates his "global" quality-of-life over the previous two days at a seven out of ten. The clinician speaking is a Palliative Care physician, and this portion of the conversation occurred close to the beginning of the consultation.

```
 1  MD:  I like to- uh- usually start out with- I have a few questions to:. (0.5) get an
 2        understanding- of: where you are and what uh: (0.8) your hopes are for
 3        this conver↓sation=Um: so- can you describe to us °your unders↓tanding°
 4        (0.5) of uh: (0.8) how you're doing right ↓now: what your hopes for care
 5        °moving forward are°? (1.8)
 6  Pt:   Well let's see °how am I feeling right ↓now.°
 7  MD:   Heh.
 8  Pt:   What to ↓say. (1.8) °Because you know°=But (0.5) I noticed the focus (0.8)
 9        with my oncologist has changed from-
10  Uk:   Sorry.
11  Pt:   ↑Trying to (1.5) treat the cancer (.) ↓right. (.) to (0.5) now (.) quality of life
12        things=Meaning, (1.0) I'm his↓tory=Okay=From that standpoint, =But now
13        we try what's ↑left of my life to make it (1.2) uh better (0.5) oh- you ↑know-
14        at least livable what ↓else minimizing these sufferings. =that sort of ↓thing.
15  MD:   Okay are ↓you (0.8) in much pain right ↑now?
16  Pt:   °No.° (1.5)
17  MD:   Is anything bothering you at all?
18  Pt:   ↑Well (0.2) I've got fluid (0.5) built ↓up (0.5) which is from the pancreas
19        and (1.0) that has to be ↓drained. (1.5) They were going to put in a catheter
20        (0.8) but I've got a temperature (0.8) a high temperature so they (0.5) didn't
21        do ↑that=Because they just drained some more fluid (0.8) But ↑that's the
22        biggest thing right ↓now. (1.2)
23  NP:   Okay (1.0) Um (0.8) so no pain right now having just had fluid drained,
24  Pt:   Yeah.
25  NP:   Okay (0.5) Um: (.) >can you tell us a little bit about< (.) uh: where you live?
26        and-
```

The physician's opening gambit in lines 1–5, a relatively standard formulation of the "presenting Palliative Care" genre (see Chapter 2), prompt the patient to reflect in line 6 on his feelings, which he proceeds to gloss with recourse to his perceptions of the changing focus of his oncologist in line 9. This suggests that how he is doing or feeling is, from the patient's own point of view, secondary in relevance to how his (non-present) oncologist has been talking. The physician is engaging in conventional "patient-centered" language: namely, eliciting the likelihood that the patient has formed hopes for this conversation and that the patient's understanding of "how you're doing", i.e., his subjectivity, is meaningfully distinct from what the clinical facts in the medical chart suggest.

The patient dodges the premise of the volley, first by repeating or recasting the phrase "your understanding of how you're doing" as "well, let's see, how'm I doing right now", and then pivoting to what he has *noticed* about others, not to how he *is* (on repetitions and their differentiated meanings, see Curl 2005; Curl et al. 2006). What the patient has noticed is a shift in attitude in his oncologist's approach to his care, which he deciphers already in line 12 as meaning that "I'm history." This is an important feature, because – as many other conversations also indicate – the patient-centered volley can often fall flat because it focuses on subjective accounts (feelings, well-being, preferences, understandings) rather than on the patient's hard-won rational work of discernment in the hospital setting – noticing, watching, waiting, and coordinating. How one is doing is often a function of what one can induce from the various patterns of clinical rounding, from the style, timbre, and genre of clinicians' voices, and from the various ways in which information is conveyed to them.

*For patients' **resistance to "patient-centered" communicative strategies**, see 2.2, 9.2, 8.5, 8.2, 8.1. For **patients' attempts to decipher the stances of other clinicians**, see 2.4, 3.5, 7.5 6.1–2, 6.5, 2.1, 6.4. For **conflicts between indirection and frankness**, see 2.1, 4.5, 5.1–3, 6.1–2, 8.3, 8.5, 9.2, 10.12.*

7.4 I'm kind of like the melancholy end of it

In the following conversation, we consider a situation that does not involve patients speaking for absent clinicians, but family members speaking for present patients, at the patients' behest. Here, again, the patient-centered communication model runs into some friction, as the patient wishes not to take responsibility for representing her "understandings", rather delegating this work, as well as the related filtering of information and decision-making, to her daughter. She wishes, in the words of the patient in conversation 2.1, to become the "silent partner" in the interaction. In the following exchange, the patient's daughter seeks to explain why and how she intends to fulfill her mother's desire to be shielded from decision-making and from the sheer volume of information that tends to vie for her attention and action in the hospital setting. We are thus interested in:

1. the ways in which patients choose to be spoken for by others;
2. how surrogates describe this responsibility; and
3. how Palliative Care clinicians respond to this division of labor.

The patient in the following conversation self-identifies as a 56-year-old white woman and as financially secure, reporting high-school-level education and no formal religious affiliation. She has been diagnosed with a stage-four cervical cancer. She believes she is "likely" to live for a year, while her clinician-rated survival prognosis is two weeks to three months. In fact, she continued to live for 5 days after this interview, drastically shorter than her expectations and significantly shorter than the clinical prognosis. She strongly ranks her end-of-life goals as "comfort over longevity" and she rates her "global" quality-of-life over the previous two days – physical, emotional, social, spiritual, and financial – at an eight out of ten. The following portion of talk occurred during the first visit of the Palliative Care team, close to the beginning of the conversation. There were ten people present for this conversation, in which the most prominent clinical speaker is an oncologist, not a Palliative Care physician. There is a Palliative Care physician in the room taking part as well, and the following sections focus on that particular Palliative Care clinician. This section begins with the daughter reviewing her relationships with the large crowd assembled.

```
1  Dt:   I've talked with every single one of you in the room. ((laughter)) hh
2  Pt:   °Yeah.°
3  Dt:   ↑Very long extensive. I- I- (0.8) I'm grasping it and, (0.2)
4  Pt:   Yeah.
5  Dt:   Like I said (0.2) there's ↑no (0.8) there is ↑no: (1.0) breaking her hope
6        (.) at ALL. ((laughter))
7  NP:   hh
8  Pt:   No.
9  Dt:   So you know (.) I'm kind of like the melancho:ly,
10 FM:   [Mm-hmm.]
11 Dt:   [ Of ]    end of it that's kind of always where (.) my (.) brain is always
12       (0.2) >preparing for the worst hope for the best< so.
13 Pt:   hh ((deep gasping breath)) °Mm-hmm°
14 NP:   °Um°
15 MD:   °All we can do is we can try to get ↑her right back into her room. =>And
16       then we continue with our conversation with ↑you,<
17 Dt:   [↑ oh    ]
18 MD:   [if that's] something that you have further (.) concerns. because I think
19       she looks=
```

20 NP: =Yeah [she's.]
21 Dt: [Quite] un↑comfortable in the ↓chair. So.

The patient's daughter, in the presence of her mother who is awake and aware throughout the interaction, takes this opportunity to introduce a division of labor by which her mother will continue to hope for a cure, while she will be responsible for the "melancholy end of it" (line 9), which she describes as her own natural disposition. In line 3, the patient's daughter intimates that she is "grasping" the gravity of her mother's clinical prognosis but, interestingly, she does not use the word "but" (at the end of line 3) to establish a contrast with her mother's stance, for whom there "is no breaking her hope." Thus the division of responsibilities is not represented here as truth versus delusion or as a tension between competing approaches, but rather as one person taking up a pragmatic stance so that the other person can maintain another, optimistic one.

1 Dt: Well ↑I don't want to keep you guys ei↓ther. °If you guys have (0.4) °°you
2   know -°°
3 MD2: It's not- one- one thing I do want to clarify ( ) I think is (.) really important
4   and- and you've alluded to as well. (0.5) ↑How: we talk with you and you.
5   (0.2)
6 FM: °Mm-hmm.°
7 MD2: And (0.2) I know there has been (0.2) um (0.2) a feeling sometimes (0.5)
8   that people are coming and saying the same (.) negative hard stuff >again
9   and again and again.< (0.5) And (0.2) what's her role (0.5) in your ↓care.
10   (.) She's a wonderful advo↓cate. (0.2)
11 Pt: Mm-hmm.
12 MD: She does a ↑great impersonation of you ↓too. ((laughter))
13 Pt: <Her ↑brain is clear.> ((laughter)) (0.5)

Having shared her plan for the division of labor in decision-making and information-management, the patient's daughter issues a pre-closing in line 1 above, anticipating that the conversation is ending, having established a new shared understanding of who will speak for whom. Another Palliative Care physician delays this closing in line 3 by re-opening the topic of frank, difficult discussion about prognosis and care planning, asking the patient to clarify exactly how *she* sees her daughter's role in the management of her care. The physician takes care in line 10 to praise the daughter's advocacy efforts, but is not entirely sure that the implicit plan the daughter outlines in the previous section about dividing the talk between hope (the patient's work) and melancholy (the daughter's work) accurately represents her mother's desires. The following exchange resolves this

concern explicitly. (As in the previous section, we are unable to analyze important aspects of eye contact and gaze direction.)

1	MD:	She- yeah her brain is ↑very ↓clear.
2	Pt:	°Right.° And so (0.5) <that's why I have no ↑qualms with her uh> (0.5)
3		<talking with ↑all of you.>
4	MD:	°Okay.° (0.5)
5	Pt:	<And (.) then she passes that on to me.> (0.5)
6	MD2:	Would you pre↑fer that? =Would you prefer that she be the one (0.2) that-
7	Dt:	I mean (.) you know if the doc- (.) I I don't ever want to take them away
8		from you to- (0.5) um, (0.5)
9	Pt:	°Right.°
10	Dt:	You know (.) to (.) ↑dampen any ↑blo::ws I it's just that um,
11	Pt:	Uh huh. (0.5)
12	Dt:	Um you know I feel: (.) sometimes (0.5) because some doctors are
13		switching in and out too: (.) so (0.2) you know I'm like why don't (.) sh- we
14		know the gist: (.) you know (0.4) you know the gist.=You have your own
15		hopes. =They (0.2) they know that (.) what's going on (0.4) and (.) you
16		know they have their num:bers: and things like that um so. (0.5) I- (.) you
17		know if anything (1.0) the (.) any repetition I can just, (0.5)
18	Pt:	<E↑radicate?>
19	NP:	Right that's all I'm-
20	Dt:	Mm-hmm.

In lines 2–5, the patient responds to the Palliative Care physician's question by
sharing her confident reliance on her daughter to pass information and decisions
on to her, describing this general procedure as something that she and her daughter have already worked out together and adhere to. This makes the physician's
cautionary follow-up interesting, because he characterizes this communication
protocol as a future aspiration, rather than an already functioning state of affairs.
The physician's abundance of caution to not unduly decenter the patient from
decision-making prompts the daughter to elucidate in 13–18 a more detailed
rationale for their ways of working. The daughter's elucidation emphasizes the
necessity of the filtering function she intends to fulfill, and this description con-
cludes with the patient's one-word, arduously produced latching contribution:
"eradicate." Whereas this word is normally associated in the hospital with "erad-
icating" cancer, like the stage-four cervical cancer she is suffering, the patient
uses "eradicate" to describe the process of reducing the mass of information she
is expected to manage as a patient. This is a striking image and strategy, which
implicitly critiques the presumptions of patient-centered communication models.

*For **clinicians' abundance of caution about patients' intentions**, see 2.4, 4.4. For **communicative divisions of labor among patients and family members**, see 2.6, 8.2, 8.3. For **metaphors of illness to characterize hospital experience itself**, see 7.6, 5.1, 5.5, 7.2. For **expressions of planned attitude management vis-à-vis hope, optimism, pessimism, etc.**, see 4.4, 10.8, 6.4, 7.1, 10.8, 10.10.*

7.5 I don't feel like I have cancer you know

Sometimes patients recount conversations with other clinicians that appear to have been Palliative Care conversations in their own right, though they may not have been conducted by specialists in Palliative Care. This following conversation prompted us to investigate the ways patients interpret prognosis-oriented messages from other specialists, and how they represent these in Palliative Care-specialized conversations later.

The patient in the following conversation self-identifies as a 70-year-old white man and as financially insecure, reporting Graduate-level education and Christian religious affiliation. He has been diagnosed with a stage-four kidney cancer. He believes he is "likely" to live for a year, while his clinician-rated survival prognosis at the time of the following consultation is three to six months. In fact, he lived 11 days beyond this consultation, i.e., shorter than clinically expected and much shorter than the patient himself expected. The patient strongly ranks his end-of-life goals as "comfort over longevity," and he rates his "global" quality-of-life over the previous two days at an eight out of ten. The clinician speaking is a nurse practitioner. Here, the patient is offering a general summary of other clinicians' assessments of his kidney cancer.

1 Pt: Well (.) from what they say: they all were in (1.0) ↑hoping that they could
2   ↑do some↓thing. (1.0) But it's (.) really too <u>late</u> (1.2) and uh (0.8) I don't
3   have any (1.0) p:ain or >anything.<I'm not (.) you know (0.5) I don't feel like
4   I have cancer °you know.°
5 NP: <u>That's</u> good.=
6 Pt: =I don't know what that's supposed to be if I ↑do. (0.8) But at this <u>point</u>
7   (0.8) I don't have any uh (2.5) <u>feelings</u> about ↓it.=I just (0.2) know that
8   (0.8) I've been going through some <u>treat</u>ments and the doctor (1.5) um (1.0)
9   said that they were not (.) gonna help ↓me.
10 NP: Mm-hmm. (0.5)
11 Pt: °So (0.2) I don't have to <u>take</u> them anymore.°
12 NP: °Mm-hmm.° (0.8)
13 Pt: And uh (2.5) there is no uh (2.5) it's the <u>not good</u>. (0.5)

14 NP: °Mm-hmm. ° (0.5)
15 Pt: More than <u>quan</u>tity they ↓say.
16 NP: °Mm-hmm.° (0.2)
17 Pt: Oh (1.0) but I don't ↑know that, (1.8)
18 NP: You don't <u>know</u> (.) which?=
19 Pt: =I don't ↑know if this (0.2) not quantity. =I might (.) outlive 'em ↑all.
20 NP: ((laughter)) .hhh There <u>is</u> a lot of un↑<u>cer</u>tainty about (0.5) about that.
21   (0.3) You know we ↑never know for cer↓tain.
22 Pt: We <u>don't</u> know. (0.8)
23 NP: [Um,]
24 Pt: [I could] get hit by a <u>bus</u> going down the street. (0.2)
25 NP: Well let's cross our fingers ↑that doesn't hap↓pen right?

At the beginning of this exchange, the patient has been asked to recount his understanding of his disease and what the other clinical teams have had to say about it.
In line 2, the patient reports "it's too late" in the indicative, not attributing it to the
clinicians with a qualifier, like "they say it's…" or "apparently." Here, it appears
the patient has already benefitted from some goals-of-care discussion from other
specialists, who have encouraged him to think about quality-of-life rather than
quantity or duration of survival. Having thought through these questions in previous conversations, he is now focused in the current exchange on the curious fact
that he does not *feel* his cancer and that the pain involved in it is minimal. This
is an example of a situation in which other specialties have prompted a patient
well about goals-of-care thinking, prior to making the referral for Palliative Care
enrollment. It is important to recognize such situations in which practitioners of
other specialties are also engaged in Palliative Care conversations, even though it
might not be a central aspect of their training or current job description. Prior to
the 2000s, when Palliative Care became a board-certified specialty, such conversations were the *de facto* purview of all clinicians throughout the hospital setting, and
this legacy of care continues, despite the establishment of a dedicated specialty.

For patients' **reflections on how they feel about their disease**, see 9.4, 4.3,
4.2, 4.1. For **patients' attempts to decipher the stances of other clinicians**, see
2.4, 3.5, 6.1–2, 6.5, 2.1, 6.4, 7.3.

7.6 It's just that he does *not* have the bedside manner

We close this chapter with one last instance in which a patient and family reflect
on the relationship between the Palliative Care approach and that of other
medical specialties. This conversation motivates us to inquire how patients and

families give voice to their values and perceptions of good clinical practice, in the course of Palliative Care decision-making discussions.

The patient in the following conversation self-identifies as an 85-year-old white man and as financially secure, reporting Graduate-level education and Christian religious affiliation. He has been diagnosed with a stage-four prostate cancer. He believes he is "very likely" to live for a year, while his clinician-rated survival prognosis at the time of the following consultation is six months. In fact, he lived 78 days beyond this consultation, i.e., shorter than both the clinical expectation and his own. The patient strongly ranks his end-of-life goals as "comfort over longevity," and he rates his "global" quality-of-life over the previous two days at a six out of ten. The following portion of talk occurred during the first visit of the Palliative Care team. The clinician speaking in the conversation is a Palliative Care physician.

```
 1  Sp:  [Well you guys –]
 2  MD:  [↑Yes. ]
 3  Sp:  Explained everything so ↑nicely. (.) And it's (0.2) ↑first time really I've
 4       had (0.5) really logical clar- (0.2) clearer (0.2) u::m (.) explanation of what's
 5       going on and ↑why they don't know? (1.5)
 6  MD:  I'm ↑glad we are:,
 7  Pt:  [Oh yeah.   ]
 8  Sp:  [Yeah you ]
 9  MD:  Being of service to (.) the both of you. (1.0)
10  Pt:  I know (0.5)
11  MD:  ↑Yes. That- that- that will be one of our (.) ↑big tasks
12  Pt:  T- take notes,
13  MD:  Yes. (1.0)      [↑U::::m- ]
14  FM:               [>I get the im]pression there'll< be ↑brief notes from
15       what they ↓said.
16  Pt:  ((laughter)) (0.5)
17  MD:  [thir↓teen seconds.]
18  Pt:  [He's got a thing.  ] over there over there and that's it.
19  MD:  ((laughter)) (1.0)
20  Pt:  >He's interesting.< He's a ↑fascinating ↓man.
21  MD:  hh Uh huh (0.5)
22  FM:  I hear he's quite smart.
23  Pt:  ↑Oh boy he's brilliant,
24  FM:  Yeah. (0.8)
```

Having expressed their gratitude about the clarity with which the Palliative Care team has described the patient's disease progression, the patient and family members enlist the team as vigilant 'note-takers' who interpret the sometimes convoluted, elliptical, or taciturn assessments of other clinicians. The group balances praise for a beloved (absent) practitioner with jokes at his expense about his unforthcoming communication style. They continue:

```
 1 Sp:  We ↑know he's an amazing <u>doc</u>tor. =And he did a beautiful (0.4) ↑thing
 2         when he came in on a <u>Sun</u>day afternoon and performed an eight and a
 3         half↓hour ope↑ration,
 4 NP:  [Mm-hmm.]
 5 FM:  [ ↑Wow ]
 6 Sp:  In an <u>emer</u>gency,
 7 Pt:  [Eight and a] half hour [operation.]
 8 Sp:                          [So I'm <u>very</u>] grateful to him,
 9 NP:  [Yes.]
10 Sp:  [It's] just that he (0.2) does not have the bedside manner (0.5) a lot of
11         doc↓tors. =↓He's <u>in</u> and <u>out</u>. (0.5) And-
12 Pt:  Like I said he's serving seven days a week twelve hours a day.=
13 Sp:  =You can't <u>ask</u> to <u>have</u> ↑everything I guess, (0.2)
14 NP:  Mm-hm
```

This and similar conversations demonstrate how Palliative Care conversations are often a treasured opportunity for patients and family members to speak openly about their experiences with other medical specialties and in the hospital in general. Among all of the other tasks at hand, they use these conversations as spaces to express assessments, critique, and gratitude toward other clinicians, often in the distant past, who have cared for them by way of a diverse range of styles, methods, and modes of communication (see Hudak et al. 2010).

For **characterizations of denial among other clinicians**, see 2.2, 10.10, 2.3, 7.6, 9.5, 8.5, 7.1, 4.2, 7.2. For **clinicians' commiseration with patients' negative experiences in hospital**, see 7.4, 5.1, 5.5, 7.2.

7.7 Insights and implications from Chapter 7

Palliative Care proceeds in a way that is often fundamentally at odds with the curative customs of the hospital, and this is reflected in the specialty's symbolic, interactional, and infrastructural relationship to other medical disciplines and personnel. The ways patients, family members, and Palliative Care clinicians thus 'ventriloquate' and 'animate' representatives of other branches of medicine is thus a complex meaning-making component of the broader arc of Palliative Care communication, and this component has come to constitute a standard rapport-building feature of the genre of the Palliative Care consultation. Through mentionings, retellings, and portrayals, patients convey rich information about their orientation to medical care as a whole and, strategically, to the various conversational practices currently underway in the interactions.

Part III: **Some Components of the Consultation**

8 Setting the table, having an agenda

In the Introduction, we discussed a number of ways Palliative Care is positioned within the overall hospital setting – symbolically, institutionally, and discursively. What tends to predominate in hospital Public Relations materials are messages of triumph, fighting, and survival, of beating the odds, and of finding strength and courage to overcome. These muscular curative discourses are powerful, and they can easily crowd out or preempt alternative lines of thinking about what can be achieved in a hospital setting, such as comfort, insight, peace, reconciliation, ease, and community. Because Palliative Care represents such an alternative body of thought – *represents* both in the sense of symbolizing and advocating – it is often the case that families and patients enter the consultation with a certain amount of wariness as to whether the Palliative Care team "has an agenda." Certainly, the last thirty years of media discourse on death and life-limiting illness have done little to disabuse families and patients of this notion.

When a Palliative Care physician or nurse practitioner meets for the first time with a patient and family, the specter that they come "having an agenda" cannot simply be dispensed with out of hand by way of a nuanced introduction of the discipline. Simply declaring that "I don't have an agenda" is a sure-fire way to convince a respective interlocutor that one doth protest too much. As we have noted in most of the conversations so far in this book, it is also likely that patients and families will enter the conversation with their own active, complex, changing, and/or hidden agendas, such that the conversation becomes one of intensive and agile "competitive framing" (Goffman 1974) on all sides.

Though some Palliative Care clinicians do claim to have no agenda whatsoever, this stance can or appear to be disingenuous. Most of the conversations discussed in this book are with patients who will ultimately have survived for a significantly shorter amount of time than they themselves expected at the time of the conversation, and one of the major recent research findings with which academic Palliative Medicine is currently contending is the problem of "prognostic discordance" – namely the often-vast gap between what patients, families, and clinicians believe about a certain disease progression (Gramling et al. 2016b). Often, clinicians strongly believe that patients have only weeks to live, while patients are certain they will live for years to come. This is of course not so much a matter of who is right, for the sake of being right, as much as it is a pattern of outcomes that shows patients and families tend to hew strongly toward received and ambient notions about the proper optimistic conduct of illness, as these are then reinforced by hospital Public Relations materials and a modern medical culture that tends to be averse to conversations about life-limiting prognoses, to inability to cure a disease, and to the event of dying

https://doi.org/10.1515/9781501504570-008

itself. And, for many of the patients discussed in this book, hospital culture is among their most primary socio-symbolic frames of reference. Whether on-and-off or continuously, they will tend to see and hear a great deal of triumphal, optimistic, curative iconography, which delivers a composite sketch of what kinds of approaches to disease and suffering are permissible, and which are somehow implicitly wayward.

Rather than "having an agenda," we suggest that Palliative Care practitioners in the best case try to "set the table" for a potentially successful collaborative consideration of the state of things. We use the vague category of "state of things" – rather than individuated formulations like "your prognosis" or "where you're/ we're at", because patients are often just as concerned about the "state of things" for their friends, spouses, or children as they may be about their own disease etiology. With this metaphor of "setting the table", we have in mind spatial, temporal, ideological, and interactional regularities that dynamically typify the genre of the Palliative Care conversation.

By **spatial**, we mean both the micro- and macro-spatial relations of hospital settings, as well as the various deictic (distal and proximal) repertoire of "heres" and "theres", including those of home, heaven, the afterlife, wellness, and the "there" of end-of-life decision-making, which is often formulated by both clinicians and family members, in the negative, as "we're not quite *there* yet." Though it would be useful for us to be able to consider the spatial relations evident in the conversations themselves, we do not have video footage that would allow for such analysis, save for the occasional conversational explicitation of those spatial relations.

By **temporal**, we mean both existential and conversational time, i.e., both the time that the patient "has" or is living, and also the sequencing and pacing of the conversation. We will remember, for instance, that the physician in conversation 2.1 announced early in the talk that "I'll ask that question often" – an utterance indicating not only that he has a principled sequential and temporal design in mind for this interaction, but also that he is willing to share the shape of that design ahead of time with the patient and family.

By **ideological**, we mean the ambient and sedimented notions that all participants bring to the talk vis-à-vis death, illness, hospitals, cures, courage, hope, and other conspicuous emotional and spiritual resources often called upon in such settings, and how those may or may not come to the surface explicitly in talk.

By **interactional**, we mean the enunciative and sequential economy of conversation generally, and clinical conversation specifically, as well as the intuitive or analytical awareness of the order of conversation – both that of the clinician and of the patient and family.

All of these factors are part of the "table" that is often set, in various ways, by a Palliative Care clinician. Other available metaphors of design, which we prefer less, are "going through some questions", i.e., allowing the conversation to be a mere interactional performance of a preexisting questionnaire, or "playing the tape to the end", which implies that the conversation is a predictable and repeatable scheme. Setting the table rather means that there are likely a number of relatively durable features immanent in a Palliative Care consultation that will arise, in unspecifiable sequence and intensity, and that it is among a physician's or nurse practitioner's primary clinical duties to anticipate these eventualities and their relationship to one another.

8.1 Is it okay to talk freely about these things?

The following conversation prompts us to inquire about the ways in which Palliative Care clinicians take on the responsibility to guide and prioritize certain tasks and topics in the conversation. We are not yet concerned in this conversation, as Barton et al. (2005) were in the ICU setting, about the substantive themes of those clinician-initiated tasks, but rather with how the clinician attempts to guide the conversation, explicitly or implicitly. We ask:

1. When is the topic of "guiding the conversation" made explicit in Palliative Care conversations?
2. Does the question of guiding the conversation seem to pertain to certain kinds of Palliative Care conversations more than others, i.e., conversations in which two clinicians are present, or where a clinician-in-training is being supported by an attending physician?
3. At which junctures does such metadiscursive recourse to "guiding the conversation" seem most potentially important or, conversely, most potentially disruptive?

The patient in the following conversation self-identifies as a 66-year-old white woman and as financially secure, reporting Associate's-level education and Christian religious affiliation. She has been diagnosed with stage-four lung cancer. She believes she will live for another year at least, while her clinician-rated survival prognosis at the time of the following consultation is two weeks to three months. In fact, she lived 11 days beyond this date, drastically shorter than her own expectations and nominally shorter than the clinical expectations. The patient is unsure whether she wishes to pursue care focused on comfort or longevity, and she rates her "global" quality-of-life over the previous two days – i.e., physical, emotional, social, spiritual, and financial quality – at a three out of ten.

The following portion of talk occurred during the first visit of the Palliative Care team. The clinician speaking is a Palliative Care physician, working together with a medical resident training in Palliative Care.

1 MD: A l:ot of what was ↑talked about earlier was (.) what's going on: (.) how
2   ill you are and what ↑might happen over time ↑right?
3 Pt: Right.
4 FM: Right.
5 MD: Is it okay? to ↑talk freely about these ↑things? (1.2)
6 Pt: She s:aid it a:ll.
7 MD: Okay you've heard all this sort of thing before?
8 Pt: °Heard it all so far.°
9 MD: Okay=Because >we just want to be prepared to do< so Doctor _____
10   detailed (0.8) your story, looked at ↑a:ll the details =and I think that's
11   very helpful =And he's gonna (1.0) help guide this conversation=I just
12   wanted to ↑offer a couple things that I think are important to focus on.
13   ((cell phone ringer music playing))

This conversation is particularly interesting for teaching purposes, because the talk is unfolding among not only a clinician and patient, but among a physician and a medical resident, referred to here in lines 9–13, and obliquely in line 1 in the passive formulation "what was talked about." The attending physician, more experienced in the genre of Palliative Care consultation and therefore likely more flexible with intuitive improvisation, steers the talk in ways that the resident does not and cannot be expected to do at this point in his own training.

Given the prognostic discordance between patient and clinician in the intake questionnaire, combined with the patient's stated uncertainty about comfort-over-longevity in care planning, the consultation is likely to be one in which the framing of conversational projects and agendas is somehow competitive from the outset. Instead of responding to the physician's bid for confirmation that it is okay to speak freely with a "yes", the family member remarks that "she's said it all," which is neither quite a response to the request but is rather a declaration that everything under the sun has already been said about her illness, and that she has no more unique contributions to make. The reason, then, that the conversation can be allowed to range "freely" on such topics as life-limiting prognosis is not that the patient is particularly willing to speak about them, but that doing so will only reiterate previous conversations. Nothing new remains to be explored; the patient is styled by her loved one to be a veteran in the conversational discourse of serious illness. The conversation continues, as the clinician recognizes a disturbing beeping noise coming from somewhere in the room.

1 MD: (1.8) Yeah >↑I know<↑Where is that coming ↓from?
2 Pt: TV and I had my [( )] on it Oh here-
3 Uk: [↑There it is]. No that's no:t it. There's a ↑speaker
4   some↓where. (0.8)
5 Pt: Yeah I know >but we always have to<
6   [find it.]
7 Uk: [I ↑got it.] Here °>let me turn that off for you guys<°.
8 MD: °Thank you.°
9 Pt: [That's what I was] looking for but ( ).
10 Uk: [You're welcome]
11 MD: [Perfect.   ] You got it. =So (.) the big question that (.) we want to help
12   ↑you decide and ↑you is (.) what (.) plan of care makes most ↓sense.
13   =↑What is it you're really looking ↓for =↑Because because I ↑kn:ow
14   that in the conversation earlier came this question of whether ↑hospice is
15   ↓right. (1.2) ↑Right?

In line 12 on page 170, the physician "want[s] to offer a couple of things that I think are important to focus on," thereby shifting the talk from the accumulation of knowledge and topics to the prioritization of choices. Interestingly, this performative gesture is interrupted by an automatic audio annoyance, a ringtone or piece of music, that continually inserts itself into the symbolic order of the room. Still in the stance of "focusing on," the physician interrupts the project of focusing on big decisions to focus on stopping the ringing in the room. These two symbolic actions act in parallel, because the family has been unable to successfully keep the alarm from going off over their time in the room, and the physician makes it his highest priority in that moment to successfully focus on that immediate task.

In this sense, the "table is set" already for these clinicians, by previous conversations with other persons, and they need to therefore reinscribe themselves into this already existing arrangement. The way the physician does this is to 1) symbolically elevate the medical resident, saying that he has "detailed your story" and "looked at ALL the details", b) then presenting his and the medical resident's position as "helping guide this conversation", c) interrupting the talk to resolve a real-time disturbance typical of hospital life, a recurring beeping sound, thus showing he is willing and able to solve immediate problems rather than hypothetical ones, and d) reconfiguring familiar, previously discussed material, of which the patient had "heard it all so far," into one "big question". This is crucial because it symbolically transforms the collected, accumulated themes of the patient's previous conversations into one superlative action.

*For patients' **resistance to Palliative Care discussions**, see 2.2, 9.2, 8.5, 8.2, 7.3. For **patients' attempts to gain recognition for their years of clinical experience**, see 3.5, 5.3, 2.3, 10.7, 5.4. For instances of **metadiscursive gestures**, see 9.2, 5.1, 5.3. For **training scenarios**, see 4.5, 2.3.*

8.2 So we're here for you

In contrast to the previous conversation, in which the clinician explicitly sought to guide and focus the talk, the clinician in this conversation seeks to create an unguided, unconstrained space in which the patient is free to express whatever his wishes may be. We are interested in this setting as a contrast to the previous one, as they show two models of how Palliative Care specialists choose to "set the table" for the talk. We ask:

1. What appear to be the advantages and disadvantages (to patients and clinicians) of open-ended, free-form discussion centered on "what you want to talk about," as contrasted with explicit attempts to "guide the conversation," as in conversation 8.1?

The patient in the following conversation self-identifies as a 58-year-old white man and as financially insecure, reporting middle-school-level education and Christian religious affiliation. He has been diagnosed with a stage-four kidney cancer. He believes he is "likely" to live for a year, while his clinician-rated survival prognosis is two weeks to three months. In fact, he continued to live for 18 days after this interview, drastically shorter than his expectations but congruent with the clinical prognosis. He moderately ranks his end-of-life goals as "comfort over longevity", and he rates his "global" quality-of-life over the previous two days – physical, emotional, social, spiritual, and financial – at a zero out of ten. The following portion of talk occurred during the first visit of the Palliative Care team, close to the beginning of the conversation. The clinician speaking in the recording is a Palliative Care nurse practitioner.

1 NP: So (2.2) we're here (0.2) for ↓you. (1.8) ↑What are the <u>kind</u> of things °you
2   wan↓ted to talk about.° (3.2)
3 Pt: Sor↓ry. ((chair scraping on the floor)) (3.2)
4 NP: ↑What- (2.2) what are some things that are con<u>cerning</u> you °at this ↓point.°
5 Sp: ↑I don't know if <u>anything</u> is right ↑now =Just (0.5) we don't know exactly
6   what's going ↑ ((inaudible)) try this new <u>thing</u>? =And until we see: what
7   happens with ↑that? (0.8) °I don't think we ↑know ↓much.°
8 NP: °Okay.°

 9 Pt: Yeah =One of the things that sort of prog↑ressive- with getting hh more
10   hh (1.0) worri↓some (.) is (1.2) uh hhhh (1.0) a:ll of this medication I'm
11   taking=I it just °seems to be° uh- and I woke up last ↑night (1.0) And I
12   had this (1.0) ho:rrible horrible tight↓ness (1.0) here: (.) and (1.2) it wasn't
13   exactly ↑nausea except that I felt that I might throw ↓up (1.0) =It wasn't
14   hhh (2) you know hhhhhh

In this conversation-initial exchange, the clinician does not, as in the previous
conversation, announce an intention to "help guide" the conversation, but rather
makes an opening volley that "We're here, for you. What are the kind of things
you wanted to talk about." The clinician's overture here is to reinforce a principle
common to most patient-centered care approaches, namely an emphatic commitment to serve the "you" of the conversation and to respond to what "you" think is
important at the time. Taking the metaphor of "setting the table," this approach
might be akin to inviting a friend to a meal and, when they arrive, asking them
whether they'd like to dine in, go out, or do something entirely different. The
burden is then on the other party to develop and express a preference, even if
they do not have one or do not wish to share it.

This is a difficult but common gambit, because it seems to evacuate responsibility for clinical discernment, focus, and prioritization, which the previous clinician in conversation 8.1 had claimed on several levels. Eliciting priorities, topics,
or preferences can be a symbolic imposition that compels patients to marshal their
energies to "set the table" themselves, or at least to imagine and then elucidate
how they would like the table to be set for them. Certainly, the relationship guest-
host-bystander is a complex one in these clinical situations, where a hospital
room may feel or become (both for the family/patient and hospital clinician) more
or less a "home" for hosting in various situations. Whereas the nurse practitioner
in 8.2 arrives as a helpful guest, the physician in 8.1 arrives as a host or at least a
facilitator, who takes responsibility for the most minute and banal aspects of the
conversational setting – including the audible disturbance that has no apparent
thematic relevance to the palliative consultation genre, at least superficially.

In line 3 above, the patient either cannot hear the nurse practitioner's
request for topics, or feigns non-comprehension with "sorry," at which point the
nurse practitioner reformulates the question as "what are some things that are
concerning you at this point." This reformulation shifts the presumed domain
under consideration from the past ("wanted to talk about", lines 1–2) to the
present ("concerning you at this point", line 4), demonstrating that the clinician understands the implicature of "sorry" to be that the patient had no topics
prepared that she would "like" to talk about. "Liking" and "preferring" are, of
course, deeply fraught and often painful propositions in Palliative Care settings,

because patients and family members are often so far from expressing anything they would like or prefer that the mere mention of these can be jarring.

The formulation "concerning you" (line 4) elicits at last a topical response from the patient's husband, who seems to dismiss the premise of the question. To view outstanding information as a "concern" is, for the family member, too much of a stretch, or does not qualify under that category. This is important, because it touches on an utterly predominant categorical schema in many of these conversations, namely the ambiguity between questions vs. concerns and between information vs. understanding. Patients are often quite sensitive when clinicians appear to have miscategorized an item under one of these schemas rather than another, or when they elicit items from one category that properly ought to belong in another.

Here, the family member is unwilling to characterize uncertainty about a treatment outcome as a something "concerning" him. It is possible to perceive this demurral as a defensive tactic, forestalling the kind of intimacy and trust required of conversations about "concerns". But it may also be a response of confusion or dismay about how the table has been set – namely, that the focus of the current conversation is to be the patient and her preferences, rather than the timely conveyance of clinical information to her. Long periods of nondisclosure, waiting, patience, impatience, and opacity – as necessarily typifies even one night's stay in a hospital, let alone a long course of equivocal and invasive curative treatments – tends to give the impression that the patient's subjectivity is not foremost in the clinical scheme of things, even if the clinicians currently involved would like this to be the case.

And yet, a full twenty seconds after the nurse practitioner's initial volley about the patient's "likes" and then "concerns" for conversation, the patient does indeed take the opportunity to express "one of the things that is sort of progressively getting more worrisome" (lines 9–10). This follows immediately on the clinician's "okay", with which she acknowledges the spouse's non-uptake of the conversational project of expressing "concerns". In a sense, it took a flat-out rejection of the initial question to make way for a repair and response to that very question. The patient, it seems, used the twenty seconds to ruminate on the mentionability of one concern that she wished to disclose: namely, the increasingly complex and extreme medication regimen that she is on. Much of Palliative Care communication is indeed designed around shoring up the mentionability of topics that patients and family members may believe to be below the bar of relevance for clinical concern.

To summarize, the sequence has been as follows: a) The clinician issues patient-centered cue, b) patient politely demurs it or cannot hear it, c) clinician reformulates question without the premise of "kinds of things you wanted to talk about," replacing it with "what's concerning you at the moment," d) her spouse runs interference, both on a and c, perhaps taking a cue from patient's polite "sorry," e) the clinician acknowledges the rebuttal and, perhaps, begins to close the conversation, f) patient, tracing these various steps, finds reason to grant the original premise elicited. Eventually the "sitting down" at the metaphorical table does indeed take place, but apparent pragmatic failure and repair must be completed first. In the next conversation, "concerns" are also addressed, but through a significantly different "table-setting."

For **patients' resistance to patient-centered communication**, see 2.2, 9.2, 8.5, 8.2, 7.3. For **family members' interventions on behalf of the patient**, see 2.6, 7.4, 8.3.

8.3 And that's to help my wife pay for stuff

The next conversation suggests that perhaps patient-centered volleys like that in the conversation-initial excerpt in 8.2 may be more successful and generative when they are preceded by a clinician-centered sequence that builds confidence in the value of clinician, thereby ratifying him or her into the community's confidence.

The patient in the following conversation self-identifies as an 80-year-old white man and as financially secure, reporting Graduate-level education and no religious affiliation. He has been diagnosed with a stage-four cancer, but has not been biopsied. He believes he is "very unlikely" to live for a year, while his clinician-rated survival prognosis is two weeks to three months. In fact, he continued to live for 34 days after this interview, which means that both his and clinicians' prognosis estimates were accurate. This person ranks his end-of-life goals as "comfort over longevity," and he rates his "global" quality-of-life over the previous two days – physical, emotional, social, spiritual, and financial – at a zero out of ten. The following portion of talk occurred during the first visit of the Palliative Care team, close to the beginning of the conversation. The clinician speaking in the recording is a Palliative Care physician, who has just finished discussing the patient's medical history.

1 MD: ↑So. =and so here we are to↓day.
2 Pt: Right.
3 MD: Um- (0.8) is >that a pretty good summary of where< things ↓are?
4 Pt: I think <u>so,</u>
5 MD: Okay, [↑One of   ]
6 Uk: [Every   ] everybody agree.

7 Sp: And also, yeah and also the-
8 Dt: Yeah. [He has ulcers.   ]
9 MD: [He's also got the ul↓cer] =Right. =which has (.) been <u>pretty</u> (.)
10   ↑rapidly getting ↓worse.
11 Sp: That's correct.
12 Dt: [Yes.]
13 Pt: [Yeah.]
14 MD: So (0.8) The other th- (0.2) other ↑tha:n (0.2) the stuff with the cancer
15   and the ulcer: =is there any other concerns you have today, =↑Pain
16   nausea vomi↓ting anything else (0.8) that I need to: (.) make sure we:
17   (.) take care of to↓day.
18 Pt: °I don't think so.°

In this exchange, the physician issues no patient-centered overtures along the
lines of "we're here for you" and does not ask the family or patient what they
want to or would like to talk about. The "concerns" that are elicited are about
anything that "I need to make sure we take care of today" (line 17). In that sense,
the physician is eliciting tasks for him to be responsible for, rather than topics
for the patient to express current feelings about. He does a spot check to see if
"that's a pretty good summary of where things are" in line 3 and how we got to
where "here we are today" (line 1). This is table-setting language in the sense
that it is preparatory, logistical, and summative and does not work in the realm
of preferences, likes, or wants. The family members are clearly satisfied with this
expediency-based approach, which seeks informational confirmation from them
rather than open topics. The conversation then continues in a more conventionally patient-centered way:

1 MD: ↑Good .hh (1.2) ↑So (1.8) wa?- the ↑next, (.) thing I want to look at is
2   what's important to <u>you</u>? (.) or to your fami↓ly. (1.2) =Going forward
3   from he:re =What are you wanting to focus on or what's imp<u>ort</u>ant. (1.0)
4 Pt: U:m (0.8) Well- extend my life (.) as ↑long as w- as we can.
5 MD: ↑Okay (1.0) >Extend your life as long as you can.<
6 Pt: Yeah. (0.8) And ↑that's – (1.2)
7 Dt: Well within <u>reason</u>,
8 Pt: Yeah within reason =And that's to help my wife ↑pay for stuff (0.5)
9   <u>Re</u>ally (0.5) Frankly.
10 MD: ↓Okay.(.hhhh) (2.2)
11 Dt: He's saying that (.) >but he's already did a DNR order yesterday and he
12   doesn't wanna< (.) um: >intubation or anything like that and he- so- <
13 Pt: ↑<u>Yeah</u> (0.3) [Don't want that but   ] -

14 Dt: [Extend his ↑life   ] like <u>this</u> but not, (0.5)
15 Pt: ↑Yeah
16 Dt: °In a <u>worse</u> condition. °

Having solicited confirmation that everything is in place and the table is set, the physician then moves to the volley of goals-of-care "focus" and "importance," which he has earned in the previous string of talk by expediently building with the family a collaborative repertoire of shared fact, i.e. a table-setting, that brings "us" to "where we are today." The patient's response is unequivocally that he wishes to focus on extending his life as long as possible, for financial reasons; it appears that his spouse receives a higher monthly financial benefit or dividend as long as he remains alive. Family members immediately undermine this asser-tion, calling attention to the counterevidence that he has completed a DNR form, preventing him from being kept on long-term life-support (see Abbot et al. 2001). All of these admissions and counter-admissions are the conversational fruit of the table that had been set previously, through a particular introduction and staging. What we notice in this arrangement is that the topics of importance to the family come more forthrightly in interaction once rapport has been built through a counterintuitively non-patient-centered sequence of expedient task-listing on the clinician's part. In the next conversation, too, the family members find these sober, logistical guided consultations encouraging.

For **clinician-centered communication**, see 2.1. For **frankness and indirec-tion**, see 2.1, 4.5, 6.1–2, 7.3, 8.5, 9.2, 10.12.

8.4 Awesome. Can I have that?

The patient in the following conversation self-identifies as a 68-year-old Asian woman and as financially secure, reporting middle-school-level education and Hindu religious affiliation. She has been diagnosed with a stage-four stomach cancer. She believes she is "unlikely" to live for a year, while her clinician-rated survival prognosis is 24 hours to two weeks. In fact, she continued to live for 4 days after this interview, which means that both her and the clinicians' prog-nosis estimate were accurate. She strongly ranks her end-of-life goals as "comfort over longevity" and she rates her "global" quality-of-life over the previous two days – physical, emotional, social, spiritual, and financial – at a two out of ten. The following portion of talk occurred during the first visit of the Palliative Care team, close to the beginning of the conversation. The clinician speaking in the recording is a medical student, who is discussing with the family members hospice as a potential next placement.

1 MS: Um: and your- and your wife is ↑right =There's this- this almost:
2 ↑gradient of: (0.5) what limitations patients set on their care =But ↑really
3 the <i↑dea> of- if we're talking about hospice- so let's focus on ↑that kind
4 of idea is: (1.2) ↑really (.) putting comfort and quality (0.5) first.
5 Sp: Right.
6 MS: And- and that means (1.2) for example not necessarily checking her
7 °heart↓rate-°
8 Sp: °Right.°
9 MS: Um: every four hours =Or her blood pressure every four hours.
10 Sp: °It would be hard for her to moni↓tor too.°
11 MS: Right. hhh And it means (0.2) not necessarily ↑having um (0.5) some
12 of these medications that people >had been on for a long time< so no
13 multi-vitamins: or -
14 Sp: °Right.°
15 MS: Or- or blood pressure medications (.) But really focusing on things that
16 (0.2) if the if _____ isn't giv:ing her? is making her uncomfortable? Then
17 °we can treat that and continue that°.
18 Sp: Can we ↑make those choices of like you know- like we don't want her to
19 not be fed (.) °we want to keep the feeding going.° (0.5) um.
20 MS: And that's some↑thing? [if -   ]
21 Sp: [And that's] you know there- you know (1.0) we
22 haven't talked about it but-
23 FM: Feeding would be: continued right?
24 MS: You mean the feeding through the tube?
25 Sp: Yeah.
26 FM: Right now the way she's taking the-
27 MS: ↑Oh thank you °thank you° (0.5) um- (0.5) it could ↓yes. =The: the thing
28 is =if the feeding is: something that's making her uncomforta↓ble (0.5) if
29 that's one of the things that triggering her nau↓sea=
30 Sp: =Right.
31 MS: Is that something that she would want to continue,
32 Sp: Right.
33 MS: So as (.) as people start to get closer to: the end of their ↓life (1.0) their
34 desire for food (0.2) goes away?
35 Sp: ↓Yeah.
36 MS: And: (.) they don't experience ↓that (.) hunger
37 Sp: that we have.↑Right ↓right =And honestly >I don't know if it's the food
38 that's making her nauseous< (.) or the drinking of water.
39 MS: Mm:

The conversation took place between a medical student and the patient's spouse, when there was a shared understanding of how close to death the patient was. There is sequentially intensive confirmation, acknowledgement, and negotiation of detail between the clinician and the patient's spouse in this string of talk above, and the level of detailed clinical speculation the medical student engages in seems to invite and encourage the family to think actively and collaboratively with her. In this sense, the conversation is a well-set table that includes many elements of a "sit-down" conversation: detail confirmation, pre-negotiation, negotiation, logistics, delegating, and so on.

```
1  Sp:    >If the drinking of ↑water< (0.8) ↑makes her ↑nauseous >but it also
2         brings her ↑comfort.<
3  MS:    Yeah.
4  Sp:    Tha:t's a tricky one.
5  MS:    An:d we would let her ↑do that.
6  Sp:    ↑Drink the water.
7  MS:    And if there was: =and if there was something else that she really
8         liked [to eat]
9  Sp:         [ right]
10 MS:    Or drink if:
11 Sp:    ↑Yeah.
12 MS:    For me? ice ↑cream?
13 Sp:    Yeah.
14 MS:    If somebody denied me ice cream I would be very upset.
15 Male:  ↓Right.
16 MS:    (h) Um-
17 Sp:    >But it might make her<But can you give her ice cream if it's gonna:-
18         =it might be ↑nice and then (.) then she feels miser↓able (0.5) because
19         she's ↓°throwing up her ice cream.°
20 MS:    We would do whatever she w:anted to-
```

In the previous section, the spouse's most emphatic question was unsolicited and formed in line 18 on the previous page: "Can we make choices of like you know like we don't want her to not be fed." This opens up a discussion of the details and scenarios of end-of-life feeding, hunger, taste, pleasure, and suffering and gives the medical student an opportunity to confidently clarify in line 20 above that "We would do whatever she wanted to."

```
1  Sp:    >Okay<
2  MS:    And sometimes? es↑pecially? people who have the (.) head and neck
3         cancers? or the cancers that affect their ability? to swallow?
```

4 Sp: Right. Mm-hmm.
5 MS: The <u>taste</u> of the (.) of whatever
6   [food it is,]
7 MS: [just the ( )]
8 Sp: Is really im<u>por</u>tant and so they can-
9   [↓Spit it out.]
10 MS: [↑Try it] °and then spit it out.°
11 Sp: So you do ( ) stuff like <u>that</u>?
12 MS: <u>Sure</u>?
13 FM: ↑<u>Awe</u>some? (0.5) Can ↑I have ↑that? [((laughter))]
14 MS: [((laughter))]
15 FM: [NO] ( ).
16 MS: So.
17 FM: >I guess I could do that myself.<
18 MS: But it's really (.) stepping back and saying what are her goals to <main<u>tain</u>
19   her> her ↑<u>dig</u>nity and her (.) her (0.2) her <u>com</u>fort as her (0.5) cancer
20   continues to progress and will <u>even</u>tually take her life.
21 Sp: I mean at this point (1.0) she had at some point talked about wanting to
22   be home for (.) only a >few <u>days</u>< (1.0) but I don't know how re<u>alistic</u>
23   that is? Heh? (0.5) An:d she-

The detailed elaboration of practical scenarios around the patient's dying process
further clarifies for the family that the rationale of Palliative Care is to follow the
wishes of the patient first, even if this involves clinical consequences that do not
on the face of them appear to promote health – i.e. that ice cream, though pleas-
urable on the lips, might cause nausea later. This sit-down sequence develops
rapport and confidence between the family member and the medical student,
leading the family member to express that some of these techniques sound
"awesome" and enviable.

For **detailed prospective descriptions of the dying process**, see 3.2, 10.1,
4.3, 3.6. For **family members' concerns about food and drink in end-of-life processes**, see 3.6, 10.10. For **characterizations of Palliative Care therapies as lux-
uries**, see 2.5.

8.5 Using the restroom is a priority in life

Frequently, the clinical team's concerted, or less than concerted, desire to guide
the conversation toward "big picture" reflection on the current state of treatment
outcomes runs at cross-purposes with the immediate priorities of the patient or

family, and this non-correspondence results in scalar discrepancies about what counts as "important" amid the various perspectives of interacting speakers. The following conversation exemplifies this dynamic in which the patient is employing several strategies to misrecognize the clinicians' conversational table-setting designs, or to reframe them for her purposes.

The patient in the following conversation self-identifies as a 56-year-old white woman and as financially secure, reporting high-school-level education and no formal religious affiliation. She has been diagnosed with a stage-four cervical cancer. She believes she is "likely" to live for a year, while her clinician-rated survival prognosis is two weeks to three months. In fact, she continued to live for 5 days after this interview, drastically shorter than her expectations and significantly shorter than the clinical prognosis as well. She strongly ranks her end-of-life goals as "comfort over longevity," and she rates her "global" quality-of-life over the previous two days – physical, emotional, social, spiritual, and financial – at an eight out of ten. The following portion of talk occurred during the first visit of the Palliative Care team, close to the beginning of the conversation. There were ten people present for this conversation, but the most prominent clinical is speaker is an oncologist, not a Palliative Care physician, though there is a Palliative Care physician in the room taking part as well. The patient is describing her current concerns, particularly as they pertain to her experiences at night in the hospital.

1	Pt:	The ↑cr:ew in the ↑evening don't want to uh- (1.0) huh (.) they don't
2		want to put me in the ↑potty chair to go to the <u>bathroom</u>. =And so (.) they
3		tried using the bed↓pan (0.5) .hhhh not for <u>pee</u>. =I can't go. =I had (0.5)
4		to force myself yesterday to use it for (0.8) 'cos I had 'em (.) uh put in uh-
5		uh- (0.8) °sup↑pository and° (.) for ↑after my um (1.2) my uh- (1.4)
6	FM:	°<u>Radiation?</u>°
7	Pt:	↓Yeah (1.5) And .hh-
8	FM:	They were-
9	Onc:	In- in- fact.=I- I know that you've been having trouble (.) ↑especially
10		in the <u>evening</u> shift with um (.) >using the <u>bathroom</u>.< =[I think that's
11		something] that we (0.5)
12	Pt:	[<u>Very</u> ↑much so,]
13	Onc:	We can address:. Um-
14	Pt:	I hope so.
15	Onc:	When ↑we- (1.0) we. =we've <u>gotten</u> together as a <u>group</u>: -
16	Pt:	°Mm-hmm.°
17	Onc:	Um you know ↑really <u>to</u>- (0.8) to make sure that everybody's on the same
18		<u>page</u>

19 Pt: ((clears throat))
20 Onc: And we have an understanding of uh (.) like the <u>big</u> picture. -
21 Pt: °Yeah.°
22 Onc: What's going ↓on.

It is clear that the patient wishes to identify a problem with the floor personnel, while the oncologist wishes to recast this as the patient "having trouble [...] in the evening shift." We see in this sequence the emergence of competitive framing (Goffman 1974) around what counts as "big picture" thinking worthy of such a large-group meeting as this. The patient is advancing a project in which the "big picture" consists of small logistical and pragmatic circumstances that can be addressed and fixed, while the clinical team wants to elicit and co-create an inductive, abstract summary of prognosis thinking. The patient's emphatic follow-up in line 14 shows that she is intent on holding the floor for her concrete "big picture" as long as possible. The talk continues with what we might call a filibuster on the patient's part, designed to fortify what she feels ought to be the main *sine qua non* big-picture topic – being able to appropriately and comfortably defecate (on turn-continuation prosody, see Auer 1996).

1 Pt: And I ↑know it's im↑portant and it's im↑perative that I (.) <u>go</u>: (1.0) um
2   (1.5) but it's <u>go</u>tten- it's ↑gotten pretty ↑<u>ba</u>d here the last three days
3   about this ↑bathroom ↓thing. =That I'm <u>al</u>most ready to not (0.8) do any
4   sup↑positories either (0.8) Just so I can at ↑<u>least</u> ↑use the ↑<u>rest</u>room,
5   0.5) 'Cos it's <u>really</u> diffi- ↑it's it's an em↑barrassment ↓thing.
6 Onc: Mm-hmm. (1.2)
7 Pt: Going to the rest↓room in a <u>pan</u>. =Especially ↑poop (0.8) <u>I'm</u> sorry. it's
8   just disgus↓ting °you know° (2.2) Um but anyway that's- I did that
9   yesterday for <u>y'all</u> so at least (1.5) I'm ↑<u>go:</u>ing. =Uh.
10 Onc: I- it's - that's important to ↓know because-
11 Pt: Yeah I <u>know</u>?
12 Onc: It's important for us to know what's important to ↓you

In line 9, it emerges that the patient is framing defecation (in a bedpan) as an item of exchange, by which she does something "for y'all," rather than – say – for herself. The oncologist then in lines 10 and 12 attempts an ostensive valorization of the patient's story, but this uptake is categorical rather than substantive, in that the clinical team collectively does not regard defecation as an important enough topic at the moment to speak about in detail. We may regard the oncologist's recasting here as an attempt to 'preempt trouble' (Chatwin 2008; Drew 1997; Koenig 2011; see also West 1984b; on evasions, see Clayman 2001). Defecation is affirmatively labeled in lines 10 and 12 as something valuable and important merely on the basis that the patient is narrating its value and importance, but shared recognition of this value does not translate into practical uptake. This imbalance and condescension is not lost on the patient, who restages her filibuster in a rather pedagogical tone that universalizes the value of defecation in the face of its apparent minimization in the current sequence thus far:

1	Pt:	Mm-hmm. Well, ((clears throat) (1.8) Using the restroom is (1) uh as we're
2		all human be↑ings it's uh: ↑priority in life you have to <u>go</u>? (1.2) And
3		um (0.8) if I could have gone to the ↑restroom? I could have gotten it <u>all</u>
4		↑out at <u>once</u>, (1.2) instead of uh what took ((door closing)) <u>place</u>? (0.5)
5		yesterday, (0.8) um- (1.2)
6	Onc:	<u>Well</u> if we-
7	Pt:	And I have to, (0.8) di↑cker with these people and I'm like– (0.5)
8	Onc:	Yeah. =so let's- <u>let's</u> spend= =I'll <u>look</u> into it this a:fternoon. =We'll
9		talk with nursing °and um° (.) just make sure that we can all come
10		across something that's -
11	Pt:	That's gonna [↑work?]
12	Onc:	[That's] agreeable and that will work.
13	Pt:	Yeah.
14	Onc:	But for ↑now? I was: (0.8) I was hoping that we could start out with um-
15		(1.2) hhh you <u>two</u> really being able <u>to</u> (0.5) if you wou<u>ld</u> (0.5) be willing
16		<u>to</u> (0.5) just-

The competitive framing here displays the non-correspondence of projects and the cross-stylistic friction at hand, and the patient is deft in her attempts to finish the sentences of the clinicians to her interactional advantage. Refocusing the conversation on what will "work" in line 12 is such a charismatic intervention on the patient's part, that the oncologist appears to feel compelled to repeat the token "work" in her response, after her preferred recasting of the presumptive shared goal of being "agreeable."

For **competitive framing**, see 2.2, 9.2, 8.5, 8.2, 8.1, 7.3. For **frankness and indirection**, see 2.1, 4.5, 6.1–2, 7.3, 8.3, 9.2, 10.12. For **complaints about absent clinicians**, see 7.5, 2.2, 10.10, 2.3, 7.6, 9.5, 7.1, 4.2, 7.2.

8.6 Insights and implications from Chapter 8

The conversations shared in this chapter demonstrate that patient-centeredness is often a much more complex endeavor than just soliciting patients' desires and opinions. Abstaining from guiding the conversation is also not a sure-fire way to make certain that patients feel recognized and respected. There may be complex discursive combinations of authority and receptivity that 'work' for certain individuals and speech communities in contexts of serious illness, while an ethos of openness and agnosticism does so for others. As Palliative Care as a medical discipline matures and trains new generations of practitioners in interactionally nuanced ways, its capacity to intricately 'set the table' for consultations with dispositionally and culturally diverse groups of patients will likewise require ongoing interactional research.

9 Knowing the history

Patients who are referred for Palliative Care consultations tend to come with extensive, complicated, and confusing "medical histories," in the material and logistical form of medical charts, referrals, insurance claims, transfers, and multiple-site treatment schedules (see also Boyd and Heritage 2006). There are often more than a handful of physicians and other clinicians actively involved in their care, most of whom do not have a reliable and customary conduit through which to communicate with each other – except the medical record. Patients, however, reasonably expect that clinicians are or should become able to assimilate and narrate this history in a more logical and coherent way than they themselves can, or at least that they can exert some rationalizing effect on the disparate pieces of institutional experience the patient has undergone. Depending on specialty, institution, technological platform, and individual clinician proclivities, medical records can be notoriously uninformative, often geared more to the purposes of receivables departments than of other clinicians' needs. Palliative Care referrals often take place without any substantive conversation having taken place with the referring physician, and Palliative Care clinicians are often left to reassemble a health history from the information provided by the record, sometimes mere minutes before entering a patient's room.

This chapter is thus dedicated to the frictions and techniques involved in acknowledging patients' and family members' reasonable expectations that a newly arrived Palliative Care clinician will have some emerging familiarity with a patient's often extensive health and treatment history. We will see in this chapter a number of strategies, rituals, and interactional phenomena that emerge from this dynamic, in which epistemic status and epistemic stance are being negotiated between veteran health services consumers on the one hand and newly arrived clinicians trained in their specialty but not necessarily well-versed in the patient's history.

9.1 I've looked at your wife's record

One reasonable presumption about the value of knowing the ins-and-outs a patient's clinical history, or "chart", would be that the more familiarity a clinician can display with the information, duration, and details of a disease history, the easier it will be to engender rapport with patients and families. We ask:
1. Should clinicians be expected to assimilate all of the various aspects of a seriously-ill person's medical history before speaking with him/her?
2. Is speaking with a seriously-ill person, without being able to account for all aspects of the medical history, bound for rapport loss?

https://doi.org/10.1515/9781501504570-009

The following conversation suggests that this is not entirely the case. The patient self-identifies as a 55-year-old white woman and as financially secure, reporting Associate's-level education and Christian religious affiliation. She has been diagnosed with a stage-four breast cancer. She believes she is "very likely" to live for a year, while her clinician-rated survival prognosis at the time of the following consultation is two weeks to three months. In fact, she lived five days beyond this consultation, i.e., drastically shorter than both her and clinicians' expectations. The patient strongly ranks her end-of-life goals as "comfort over longevity," and she rates her "global" quality-of-life over the previous two days – i.e., physical, emotional, social, spiritual, and financial quality – at a five out of ten. The following portion of talk occurred during the first visit of the Palliative Care team, represented here by a Palliative Care nurse practitioner.

1 NP: And that =you know I've ↑looked at (.) I've looked at your wife's record.
2   =↑Oh my <u>God</u> -
3 Sp: °Yeah.°
4 NP: She's been °<u>fighting</u> this° since 200<u>4</u>.
5 Sp: Right. >A lot going <u>on</u>< yeah?
6 NP: A lot going on=She's been (.) getting (.) <u>really</u> good reasonable
7   treatments.
8 Sp: Mm-hmm.
9 NP: °You guys have been fighting really <u>hard</u>.°
10 Sp: ↓Mm-hmm.
11 NP: I know about the <u>last</u> three weeks =I <u>heard</u>-
12 Sp: ↓Yeah.

What becomes clear in lines 1–4 is that reiterating all of the details of a patient's medical history is not the only way to demonstrate adequate appreciation for the complexity of her condition and past experiences. The nurse practitioner's affective stance in line 2 does this symbolic work by expressing intense surprise at the accumulated experience the family has sustained with this illness. Sharing that surprise is enough in this sequence to position the nurse practitioner both as a respectful newcomer engaging in appropriately inarticulate expressions of emotion around arrival into an unknown context and, at the same time, as a knower who can intuitively grasp the scope of the family's experience. From this perspective, it is not always the case that "the more, the better" when displaying familiarity with the treatment history. Sometimes affective stance is better, and more efficient, at achieving the work of any epistemic status-design the clinician is aiming to effect.

*For **clinician expressions of surprise**, see 4.1. For **clinician expressions of admiration of patients**, see 3.4, 4.1, 9.3, 5.5.*

9.2 I'm really not interested in what you have to say

Often, upon referral, a patient or family member begins the Palliative Care conversation by expressing frustration about what they see as discrepancies in the order of operations in intergroup clinical conversation. That is, they cannot appreciate the rationale for a Palliative Care conversation *at this moment*, when representatives from another medical specialty have yet to round back to the room with desired information that might make them more prepared for such a conversation. Sometimes this unwillingness is an expression of accumulated frustration about hospital communication pathways and procedures generally; other times it is a way of objecting to the very idea of a Palliative Care referral when other curative specialties have yet to deliver expected clinical results or assessments. The following conversation plays out a number of these dynamics. We ask:

1. Should a Palliative Care consultation be timed in specific relation to when other clinical specialties round?
2. Is this a logistical possibility?
3. When coordination of information is not possible, what expectations among patients and families tend to be thwarted, and how is this expressed?

The patient self-identifies as a 75-year-old Black woman and as financially secure, reporting Associate's level education and Christian religious affiliation. She has been diagnosed with a stage-four lung cancer. She believes she is "likely" to live for a year, while her clinician-rated survival prognosis at the time of the following consultation is two weeks to three months. In fact, she continued to live for 123 days after this consultation, i.e., longer than clinicians expected, but shorter than the patient expected at the time of consultation. The patient ranks her end-of-life goals as "comfort over longevity," and she rates her "global" quality-of-life over the previous two days – physical, emotional, social, spiritual, and financial – at a six out of ten. The following portion of talk occurred during the first visit of the Palliative Care team.

1 Pt: And ↑she ( ) I'm ↑really not interested in what you have to ↓say <until
2   they give me> more of a- more of an ↓explanation.
3 NP: ↑Okay.
4 Pt: Of where they uh what's <u>wrong</u> with me ↓now. with what's <u>happen</u>ing °in
5   my lungs.°
6 NP: ↑Fair enough,

```
 7  Pt:   °Is ↑that good?°
 8  NP:   That's [fine.]
 9  Pt:          [Okay.]
10  NP:   Are ↑they, are ↑you (1.2) ↑were they- did they say they would come back
11         ↑in today? or have they already been
12         [   around?      ]
13  Pt:   [ Oh I'm sure    ] they'll- they've been in several ↓times =and I'm sure
14         somebody's (0.5) °↓coming back.°
15  NP:   ↑So (0.5) >I can leave it at ↑that< and we can check: back in with ↑you
16         to kind of see. (0.5)
17  Pt:   Okay.
18  NP:   You know=where thi[ngs are]
19  Pt:                     [do they?]
20  NP:   >and if you have< any ↑questions.
21  Pt:   ↓Okay.
22  NP:   We <we're not here to be a b:urden>. We jus:t- we want to help if there's
23         a way that we can [help.]<
24  Pt:   [Okay.]
25  NP:   <Okay?>
```

This is a setting in which the patient clearly objects to the sequence of rounding and is unwilling to engage in a Palliative Care conversation with the nurse practitioner until she feels that she has been able to access the information she needs from other clinicians (see Carr 2006). The nurse practitioner essentially accepts this stance, but attempts in lines 20 and 23 above to re-illustrate an abstract willingness to help. This sequence leads the patient's daughter to confront the nurse practitioner's rationale around such willingness to help, and the overall coordination-of-care procedures that underlie it. The interaction continues:

```
 1  Dt:   >Can I just ask a question< [about ]
 2  NP:                               [↑Sure.]
 3  Dt:   your role?
 4  NP:   ↑Yeah.
 5  Dt:   in this whole ↑thing:?
 6  NP:   ((cough))
 7  Dt:   And it- it just seems to me that- okay you're °coming in to talk to the patient.°
 8  NP:   °Mm-hmm.°
 9  Dt:   °Uh my° mother about her ↓symptoms. (1.0) Wouldn't ↑you like connect
10         with the other ↑doctors to talk about what her issues ↑are? =Do you do
11         that as ↑well? [Or what do you do?]
```

12 NP: [↑We- we ↑do.] We <u>do</u> do that. ↑Um I- you know before I
13   came in I looked at her ↑chart and kind of <u>saw</u> the the <u>issues:</u> that you
14   brought you >into the hospital,< and: the things: that they've <u>been</u>: (0.5)
15   ↑doing: to try to alle<u>viate</u> those <u>issues.</u> =I know you went down for a
16   ↑procedure ↓to<u>day</u>? (0.5) Um: if if there's ↑specific questions =we'll often
17   speak >↑with the <u>doctors</u>?< and we- we do try to do that (.) when we have the
18   chance. Uh ↑you just mean because I'm asking her all the <u>question:s</u>? Or. (2.0)
19 Dt: >↑You answered my question.< (0.2)
20 NP: Okay. (1.0)

The family member is cordially attempting to challenge the nurse practitioner
to demonstrate coordination and management of information between her and
the other clinicians and specialties, and is questioning the purposefulness of the
current consultation, if such coordination among the clinical teams has been less
than optimal thus far. The daughter's response in line 19 demonstrates that she,
unsatisfied with the response that the clinician provided, has decided to with-
draw any further discussion of the topic. This is clearly a moment of rapport-loss,
though one nearly necessitated by the patient's earlier statement "I'm really not
interested in what you have to say until…" Here we see how intimately rapport in
conversation is dependent on other coordination-of-care preparations and on the
conduct of organizational behavior prior to the consultation visit, without which
a consultation is often perceived as moot by the patient and family.

For instances of **rapport loss**, see *5.3*, *5.2*. For **frankness and indirection**, see
2.1, *4.5*, *6.1–2*, *7.3*, *8.3*, *8.5*, *10.12*. For **frustration with institutional protocols**, see
5.3, *2.4*, *9.3*, *9.5*.

9.3 Are you familiar with how long she's been going through this?

When a patient or family member is skeptical as to whether a clinician is
well-informed about the details of their health and treatment history, this uncertainty often does not surface immediately or explicitly. We ask:
1. How do family members express doubt or frustration with a clinician's apparent unfamiliarity with the details of a patient's health history?
2. When such confrontations occur, how can clinicians best respond?

In the following conversation, the patient's spouse's silence turns out to be
an expression of skepticism (see Bolden 2010), which then comes to light in a
sudden spot-check that takes the clinician somewhat off-guard and prompts a

series of repair actions. The patient in the following conversation self-identifies as a 58-year-old white woman and as financially insecure, reporting middle-school-level education and Christian religious affiliation. She has been diagnosed with a stage-four kidney cancer. She believes she is "likely" to live for a year, while her clinician-rated survival prognosis is two weeks to three months. In fact, she continued to live for 18 days after this interview, drastically shorter than her expectations but congruent with the clinical prognosis. She moderately ranks her end-of-life goals as "comfort over longevity," and she rates her "global" quality-of-life over the previous two days – physical, emotional, social, spiritual, and financial – at a zero out of ten. The following portion of talk occurred during the first visit of the Palliative Care team, close to the beginning of the conversation. The clinician speaking in the recording is a Palliative Care nurse practitioner, and the patient is reporting what the oncology team had told her prior to the consultation.

1	Pt:	↑Clearly the <u>cancer</u> is gro↓wing (1.2) And it seems to be growing much
2		· quickly than I'd an↑ticip<u>ated</u>.=Uh: (0.5) because it's always grown very
3		slowly,
4	NP:	°Mm-hmm.°
5	Pt:	Uh: hhh (1.2) He's got this <u>new</u> drug. (1.0) which uh: hhh (1.2) as soon as
6		they-=I get the <u>port</u> in <u>prob</u>ably either tomorrow or (0.2) ↑Thursday those
7		we'll have the °first chemo treatment° and then I <u>have</u> a chemo °treatment
8		every ↓month.° (1.5)
9	NP:	°Okay. °
10	Pt:	Um hhhh (0.8) and uh you know (1.0) they'll hhh monitor things to see
11		whether it's ef↓fective.=If it's <u>not</u> effective he has: (1.0) a couple of other
12		ideas: (1.2) ↑One is to go back to a drug °that's been effec↓tive° (0.5) for
13		me in the <u>past</u> which is ↑Taxol. =But I ↑think there's another °possible
14		drug that I haven't taken° and I ↑think hhh (0.8) if ↑those °do work we're
15		pretty well at the end of the ↓line.° hhh (2.0)
16	NP:	°I think so.° ((whispered)) <u>Did</u> he ↑talk <u>about</u>: (2.0) some of the (1.8)
17		b:<u>ur</u>dens (1.5) some of the <u>side</u> effects?
18	Pt:	We haven't ta- talked about it yet=°The nurse practitioner is gonna° (.)
19		bring me the lis:t to↓day. hhh
20	NP:	°Okay.°
21	Pt:	He said °I wouldn't lose my hair.° .hhhh
22	NP:	<u>And</u> you ha↓ven't yet.
23	Pt:	↑No. (1.5) hhh
24	NP:	That's a ↑tough <u>one</u>?
25	Pt:	°Mm-hmm. ° (7.0)

26 NP: Yeah. =↑So (.) what <u>we</u> know (0.8) is that (2.0) you know. =you- you felt
27   it °before when you had chemotherapy° (.) um (0.8) as <u>well</u> as (.) being a
28   <u>toxin</u> (.) a <u>poison</u> against (.) the <u>cancer</u> (1.0) it ↑also is a ↓toxin against
29   (.) the ↓<u>body</u>. (1.0) °Um°
30 Sp: A-are you fa<u>mili</u>ar with (.) how long↑ she's been <u>going</u> through <u>this</u>?

Silent for most of the interaction thus far, the spouse appears to take some umbrage at the clinician's epistemic status design in lines 26–29, where she attempts to summarize what "we know" about the ambivalent nature of chemotherapy. The umbrage-taking, an on-record positive face-threat toward the nurse practitioner, results in the clinician undertaking emphatic repair of her own face, along with a shower of praise for the patient/family's accomplishment:

1 NP: ↑Yes I ↑<u>am</u>.
2   [Yes. ↑<u>Absolutely</u>' it's]
3 Sp: [Okay, Because °I just don't know how much-]°
4 NP: In↑credible.
5 Sp: Yeah.
6 NP: Yeah,
7 Sp: °And it was o↑varian as well as uterine cancer going on more than 22
8   years ago.° =Yeah.
9 NP: It's ↑<u>fabulous</u>?
10 Sp: Yeah.
11 NP: ↑So you- you know-
12 Pt: Right?
13 NP: You know (.) how you <u>feel</u> °with the chemotherapy°. =U:m (.) s:o? (1.8)
14   we always want to ↑think about (4.5) any treatments that we <u>do</u>. (2.0) the
15   <u>benefit</u> (0.5) versus potential ↓harm.
16 Sp: °Okay.°
17 NP: Of the treatment.

Unlike in conversation 9.1, where the nurse practitioner's preemptive formulation early on in the conversation demonstrated *affective* familiarity with the intense and complicated history of treatment, the clinician in the current conversation did not pursue that form of recognition early on in the conversation, resulting ultimately in this moment of face threat and repair, in which she needed to respond with a repeated, emphatic repair in lines 2, 4, and 9.

   For **clinicians' emphatic admiration of the patient's history**, see *3.4, 4.1, 9.1, 5.5*. For **meaningful silences**, see *2.3, 3.3, 6.3*.

9.4 This adventure you've been on

Often patients and family members appreciate the use of metaphors to describe their treatment history, whether that metaphor draw on ironic, comic, poetic, or laudatory resources in language. In the following excerpt, we find an exchange between a patient and a Palliative Care clinician, in which the patient's treatment history is described as an "adventure." We ask:

1. What kinds of metaphors about illness and survival tend to be quite well received by patients suffering serious illness?
2. What level of humor is appropriate in such cases?

The patient in the following conversation self-identifies as a 73-year-old white woman and as financially insecure, reporting high-school-level education and Christian religious affiliation. She has been diagnosed with a stage-four lung cancer. She believes she is "likely" to live for a year, while her clinician-rated survival prognosis is three to six months. In fact, she continued to live for 63 days after this interview, drastically shorter than her expectations and significantly shorter than the clinical prognosis as well. She strongly ranks her end-of-life goals as "comfort over longevity," and she rates her "global" quality-of-life over the previous two days – physical, emotional, social, spiritual, and financial – at a five out of ten. The following portion of talk occurred during the first visit of the Palliative Care team. The clinician speaking is a Palliative Care nurse practitioner.

```
 1  NP:   ↑So I've looked through your chart and- =and so I think I have a ↑fairly
 2         good idea of kind of (.) the ad↑venture <that you've been on::> (0.5)
 3         [My unders- hh ((laughter)) ]
 4  Pt:   [↑That's a good way to put it.]
 5  NP:   Well it could be a good adventure or a ↑bad
 6         [adventure so -]
 7  Pt:   [Yeah.    ]
 8  NP:   I leave that to your discretion. ((laugh)) hhhhh
 9  Pt:   ↑Right,       [I'm always up ]
10  NP:                 [But I underst- ]
11  Pt:   for ↑good adven↓ture.
12  NP:   ↓Sure (0.5) I understood you've come to the hospital on: ↑Monday
13         because you were having (0.5) more ↑pain?
14  Pt:   ↓Yeah.
15  NP:   And um (0.5) some trouble with- w-were you having trouble ↑breathing?
16         (1.0)
17  Pt:   .hhhhhh it's like (.) when I um (2.5) >get up in the morning.<
```

18 NP: °Mm-hmm.°
19 Pt: And the <u>pain's</u> there. (2.5) Or (.) when: (0.5) I don't know (1.0) Now it's like
20   >when I go to the bathroom,< (0.5) .hhhhh (1.0)
21 NP: Then it <u>hurts</u> and you get up and move? (0.8)
22 Pt: Y:eah (0.5) well no, that I get out of b:reath.

This conversation exemplifies how patients frequently enjoy participating collaboratively with clinicians in creating metaphors that can account for the shape and nature of their disease, its treatment, and their survival thus far. Whereas one might assume that "adventure" is a less than apt image for contending with lung cancer, the patient appears in line 9 to join in the development of the metaphor and to creatively elaborate on her role within it.

For **metaphors of illness and survival**, see 3.2, 10.1, 4.3, 8.4. 3.6.

9.5 You've got this all wrong

The following conversation shows a situation in which it is ultimately important for the patient to be able to have an opportunity to correct the account of the history that the clinician provides, and in doing so also to correct any lingering misinformation that she perceives as persistent in her recent care. We see in this exchange the value of explicitly encouraging patients to correct clinicians' assessments and understandings, prompting them to express more of their experience than they otherwise might. We ask:

1. Is it of benefit for patients and families when the clinician humbles herself and describes her own fallibility?
2. How can a clinician's willingness to be corrected by patients or family members be expressed early on in a consultation?

The patient in the following conversation self-identifies as a 68-year-old white woman and as financially insecure, reporting Associate's-level education and Wicca spiritual affiliation. She has been diagnosed with a stage-four lung cancer. She is unable to estimate her own prognosis, while her clinician-rated survival prognosis is two weeks to three months. In fact, she continued to live for 15 days after this interview, drastically shorter than her expectations and significantly shorter than the clinical prognosis as well. She is unsure whether she prefers "comfort over longevity," and she rates her "global" quality-of-life over the previous two days – physical, emotional, social, spiritual, and financial – at a six out of ten. The following portion of talk occurred during the first visit of the Palliative Care team. The clinician speaking is a Palliative Care physician.

1 MD: What I'm <u>wonder</u>ing is- is um (0.5) >Actually you've mentioned that you
2   you guys had a <u>good</u> conversation but it was a little bit.=it was a little bit<
3   <u>tiring</u> after a ↑while, (0.5) Um (0.5) and I'm would it be help<u>ful</u> if I told you <u>my</u>
4   understanding of ↑things? (0.5) and you can correct me if I'm ↑wrong? (1.0)
5 Pt: ↑Yeah: go ahead why ↓not.
6 MD: ↑O:r if you prefer you can tell -
7 Pt: [↑Nah: you?   ]
8 MD: [You can tell   ] (5.0)
9 Pt: ↑Go for: it.
10 MD: Okay. =°Right on° (0.8) So (.) um (0.8) my understanding is that you-
11   you have a- a ↑cancer that you've known about for- for a ↑relatively
12   short period of ↓time,=um that you and that you ↑tried a round
13   of chemo↑ther:apy, (0.8) and that (0.2) you're no ↑longer using
14   >chemotherapy because it hasn't been help↓ful< (1.0) And that you came
15   into the <u>hospital</u> this time with abdominal ↑<u>pain</u>? (0.8) <u>Is</u> that ↑right? (1.0)
16 Pt: The ↑<u>chemo</u> was help↑ful.
17 MD: It <u>was</u> helpful. =Okay.
18 Pt: >Wait a minute. <You've got this whole thing <u>wrong</u>.
19 MD: Okay (0.5) >Please correct me.<
20 Pt: I (0.8) got ↓sick (1.5) I went (0.5) to get-(0.5) my <u>doctor</u> has been ↓bugging
21   me. (1.0) to get a col:<u>onos</u>↓copy (1.5) So I finally gave in: and so okay I'm
22   going to get this ↓<u>done</u> (0.8) So I went up the (0.8) and uh (2.5) to get this
23   <col:onoscopy> (1.2) And (.) I took a <↑CAT scan> (1.0) and my <u>stomach</u>
24   wasn't feeling ↓right=I knew that there was something sc:rewed ↑up in
25   there (1.2) So I said okay I'll go have this ↓thing (1.5) So ↑I <u>went</u> (0.2) And I
26   took this <CAT scan> (0.8) and (0.5) they said <we'll get <u>back</u> to ↓ya> (0.8) I
27   said okay=So the <colonoscopy was scheduled for> (.) the twenty<u>ninth</u> (1.2)
28   ↓So (0.5) I'm <u>waitin'</u> I went on the eigh<u>teenth</u> (0.5) to for the CAT scan (1.8)
29   So, (1.2) the (1.2) the- (1.8) for a ↑week I ↑waited for these guys to call me
30   <u>back</u> and (0.5) and s:ay something was wrong with my s↑tomach because
31   I <u>knew</u> something was going <u>on</u>? (0.8) I could <u>feel</u> it (0.5) ↑Plus I hadn't (.)
32   taken a <u>crap</u> in a month. (1.2) The ↑two months I did not (0.5) <u>poop</u>, (0.2)
33   No bowel movements (0.2) and I said this isn't right. =Something's ↑wrong
34   <u>here</u>. (2.0) So I turned around and (0.5) I called up the twenty-fourth at (.)
35   about nine o'clock in the <u>mornin'</u> (0.5) and said ↑hey (.) did you ↑fi:nd
36   any↑thin'? (0.8) In this CAT scan? (0.5) 'Cos my stomach <really really hurts>
37   (0.5) And (0.8) I'm wondering if there's something going >↑on in there< (1.5)
38   Well (0.5) I waited all day until <u>four</u> o'clock (0.8) and finally called me back
39   and said ↑oh you may have <u>fluid</u> on your stomach (0.5) Go in the hospi↓tal
40   (1.0) So I went to _____ (0.5) and they did a paracen↑<u>tesis</u>? (0.8)

What we find most remarkable about this conversation is that the Palliative Care physician's initial invitation for the patient to correct any wrong information he conveys appears to allow the patient space to enfranchise herself to do precisely that – not only once, but in three substantive instances in lines 17 and 19, but also in line 35, when she recounts having intervened on her own behalf when some aspect of her treatment did not 'feel right'. This sequence reminds us that it can be very valuable interactionally for a clinician to humble her/himself through the prospective scenario of eventually being corrected by the patient, when something is not perceived as accurate. Offering correction as an interactionally appropriate tool in Palliative Care conversations can go a long way to fostering engagement in the interaction, and undoing the epistemic imbalances typical of hospital settings.

For **clinician self-humbling,** see 2.6. For patients' **grievances about other absent clinicians,** see 7.5, 2.2, 10.10, 2.3, 7.6, 8.5, 7.1, 4.2, 7.2. For patients' **grievances about institutional protocols,** see 5.3, 2.4, 9.3.

9.6 Insights and implications from Chapter 9

Under current institutional conditions, it is unlikely that clinicians will suddenly find more time to review and assimilate all of the elements of their referred patients' complex and lengthy health histories. Often these histories (and their paper trails) are difficult to reconstitute even when clinicians may have been given ample time to do so. As these conversations suggest, however, there are ways that clinicians can achieve a level of authentic and holistic recognition of the experience of the patient's history that expresses a commitment to what Ellen Barton has called a "situated ethics" in Palliative Care (Barton 2006; see also Barton 2007b; Mularski and Osborne 2001; Solomon 2005).

10 Prognosis and prognostication

Seriously-ill people and their doctors from various medical specialties often have no proper forum to talk – or talk meaningfully – about clinical expectations for how long they might live, what the forthcoming course of illness may entail, what may happen as death nears, or how available medical treatments might improve or worsen any of these experiences (Gwande 2014; Lamont and Christakis 2001). For patients who indeed prefer not to take part in any decisions regarding their treatment choices as the end of their life approaches—i.e., those who wish to sustain the stop-the-disease-at-all-costs *status quo* even when actively dying, and who would not find it helpful to talk about "what to expect" from their illness—such customs or cultures of prognostic avoidance may not be problematic or unwelcome (Gramling et al. 2013a; Gramling et al. 2013b; Gramling et al. 2013c; Jones and Beach 2005; Lamont and Christakis 2001).

We begin this chapter with a range of mini-excerpts that exemplify various stances patients in our study have taken up toward prognosis. As exemplified in excerpt 10.1 below, many people consider prognosis information important for contemplating medical treatments.

10.1 I'd rather enjoy everyday

1 Pt: To be honest if I've only got 3 to 6 months to go I don't want any chemo
2   or radiation because if I'm just going to get a few extra weeks then I'd
3   rather enjoy every day that I have

Most people in the United States express preferences for end-of-life care that favors comfort and relief of stress over longevity (Hamel et al. 2017). Most also, however, have perceptions about cancer prognosis that are far more optimistic than what their oncologists believe to be likely (Gramling et al. 2016b) and choose invasive and ineffective treatments that they mistakenly believe can cure them (Weeks et al. 2012). And yet, most also experience substantial emotional/existential suffering from uncertainty about what to expect from their illness (Gramling et al. 2017) and prefer physicians to be forthright with them about prognosis in advanced illness (Hamel et al. 2017).

Indeed, Palliative Care conversations about prognosis often begin with, or otherwise include, patients and families sharing how challenging they have found attempts to engage their other doctors in conversation about prognoses. Sometimes this difficulty manifests in patients feeling that their physicians were overly ambiguous (10.2), unwilling (10.3), or reluctant (10.4) to estimate how long they might live:

https://doi.org/10.1515/9781501504570-010

10.2 He left it open-ended

1 Pt: But that was the whole thing. See, Dr. _____ just basically came in after
2   you talked to Dr. _____ and then just told me well, you've pretty much
3   got from now until whenever.
4 MD: He left it open-ended.
5 Pt: Oh, he left it WAY open-ended.

10.3 He is not going to forecast a mortality

1 Pt: He just basically said he did not feel surgery was helpful. And he is not going
2   to forecast a mortality.

10.4 He would never give us a time

1 FM: And Dr. _____ in [town] would never give us a time. _____ asked him
2   100 times and he wouldn't, said he didn't know. But the doctor in
3   Connecticut said, resisted but said, 'You know probably 6 to 18 months,
4   and he said _____ you've already gotten through 6 months...'

How we arrived at this modern medical culture of prognostic avoidance is not entirely clear, but it has at least some roots in the meteoric rise of our ability to diagnose, treat, slow, and cure disease over the past century. In the 1890s, for example, physicians-in-training would find equal space allotted, in the chapter on pneumonia in their textbook *The Principles and Practices of Medicine* by William Osler, to the three traditional pillars of medicine: diagnosis, prognosis and treatment (Christakis 1997). Over the following century, discussion of prognosis eroded to complete absence in the 1980s edition of the same textbook. In the interceding decades, we cultivated both an economic model of health care that paid hospitals and doctors quite well for diagnostic tests, invasive procedures (e.g., surgery, injections, dialysis) and longshot cure-oriented interventions (e.g., chemotherapy in advanced stages of cancer) but paid them relatively poorly for spending time listening to or talking with patients. Thus, modern physicians are provided little education about prognosis, nearly no role-modeling about how to talk about it, no or scant time to spend with patients overall, and strong incentives to focus on curative procedures.

In parallel, we developed complementary pressures that made it hard for modern physicians to tolerate almost any degree of diagnostic uncertainty.

Successful malpractice claims in the latter 20th century punished physicians for doing too few diagnostic or therapeutic procedures (and, thus, "missing" a potentially curable illness) rather than doing too many (and, thus, causing suffering related to "over-medicalization"). These cure-and-certainty expectations combined with the information explosion of medical science to create a battery of sub-specialists, many focused on one organ or one disease. "Hope" in such sub-sub-specialty-driven medicine balances magnificently, albeit precariously, on the philosophical claim that the disease of interest can be prevented, eliminated or otherwise controlled to avoid death. Indeed, we see tangible footprints of this ethos in 10.5 below, during an exchange between the Palliative Care physician and wife of a patient who is dying in the hospital on the heart failure specialty unit. The patient has advanced cancer that has been resistant to anti-cancer treatments. He is unconscious and multiple organs in his body are irreversibly failing. He has been receiving chronic life-support for more than five years from a mechanical "ventricular assist device" (VAD) that pumps blood through his body, because his severe heart failure rendered his native heart almost completely ineffective. They are preparing to turn off the VAD, to prevent symptoms of shortness of breath and allow him to die.

10.5 He's dying from the cancer really

1 MD: He's dying from the cancer, really, which makes everybody here feel
2   really good.
3 Wife: Yes, yes (laughter)

The physician's statement, both compassionate and ironic, describes a specialized medical culture that somehow "feels good" that a person who is dying will ultimately die from some other specialty's disease. Patients and families – often struggling amid these unimaginable, confusing, and terrifying moments of suffering – can occasionally feel these strange inter-specialty face-saving undercurrents. When the physician names the irony during a tender moment of connection above, it appears to provide some release for the patient's wife who apparently had been noticing this. Such a "hope equals cure equals cure-focused treatment" equation can become a patient-physician-family covenant of sorts, leading to what some have described as a "necessary collusion" in prognostic avoidance (Heft 2005) when treatments are not working any longer. (Note that the exchange above is analyzed in greater detail in 5.5.) As exemplified in 10.6 below, abdicating this *modus operandi* can be shocking for patients and families, sometimes leading to feelings of abandonment.

10.6 He threw in the towel

1 Pt: Six weeks ago he threw in the towel.
2 MD: Okay.
3 Pt: He found out that I was not doing well with that round of chemo. And he
4   was just like, You're done.
5 MD: Okay.
6 Pt: And that's what I told Dr. _____. I said well I'm not-
7 MD: How did that make you feel when he said, You're done?
8 Pt: I just told him, I said, I'm not done.

This state of affairs, often arising from communication failure in other specialty settings, sets a complex scene for Palliative Care consultations, where participants communicate about prognoses in nearly all conversations to one degree or another (Gramling et al. 2013c). The near omnipresence of prognostication in Palliative Care consultations supports the growing realization that modern medicine's avoidance of prognosis communication has created a simmering need, which has fast become a niche that Palliative Care fulfills. Indeed, improved understanding about prognosis (Temel et al. 2011) and alleviation of distress relating to prognostic uncertainty (Gramling et al. 2017) appear to be two key mechanisms by which Palliative Care ultimately improves quality-of-life for people with advanced cancer (Temel et al. 2010). Rather than attempt to cover the full landscape of prognosis disclosure and discussion in Palliative Care consultations – a topic that deserves a book-length study of its own – we focus in the remainder of the chapter on some examples that highlight primary aspects of talking about the future in advanced illness.

As we outlined in the Introduction, each participant in the parent study from which these data emerge were also asked the following questions prior to the Palliative Care consultation: "Over the past two days, how much have you been bothered by uncertainty about what to expect from the future course of illness?" Response choices included "Extremely", "Quite a bit", "Moderately", "Slightly", and "Not at all". Given their particular salience for these examples, we include these data in the descriptions below.

10.7 I am the two percent

We revisit here a conversation discussed in Chapter Six under the aegis of code-mixing, here from the perspective of prognostic discussion. The patient identifies as a 61-year-old woman with stage-four pancreatic cancer who holds a graduate degree and describes herself as Christian and financially insecure. She reports believing that she is likely to live for a year or longer, but is also extremely bothered by prognostic uncertainty. She prefers a comfort over longevity treatment focus, if faced with such a tradeoff in the last months of her life. She rates her overall quality-of-life as 1 out of 10. The Palliative Care nurse practitioner with whom she is talking estimates that the patient is likely to die within 3 months of this consultation. We do not know how long the patient lived, because she was alive at the end of the six-month follow-up period.

1 NP: [Yeah.   ] (0.8) Yeah you've been through a lot.(2.2)
2 Pt: I don't want to die. (0.5)
3 NP: No.
4 Pt: Don't want to die. (0.2) So the reason I keep asking question
5   (0.2) I don't want to die. (0.5)
6 NP: And you seem like a very very strong woman.=So- (1.0)
7 Pt: I'm very [positive.   ]
8 NP: [You're doing every]thing. =yep
9 Pt: I'm very positive.
10 NP: I think that's the best medicine right there. (1.0) I can tell. (1.0)
11 Pt: He said (0.2) you have a tough cancer. (1.2) Survival rate is only (3.2) one
12   year (0.2) the most. (1.2) And only two percent can make that. (0.2) I told
13   him (0.8) straight to his eyes (0.2) I said Doctor I'm the two percent.

In his book *Staring at the Sun: Overcoming the Terror of Death*, the existential psychologist Irvin Yalom suggests that "Self-awareness is a supreme gift, a treasure as precious as life. This is what makes us human. But it comes with a costly price: the wound of mortality. Our existence is forever shadowed by the knowledge that we will grow, blossom, and, inevitably, diminish and die" (Yalom 2009: 2). In line 4–7, the patient quite eloquently and efficiently demonstrates that fear of dying is a tangible source of her suffering.

Uncertainty can be defined as "knowing that we don't know" (Han et al. 2011). Predicting how long a person will live is, at some level, *always* unascertainable. Even amid mounting experience that therapies are not working, uncertainty offers the very space for possibility – even longshots. Indeed, believing that we can beat the odds is a cherished, celebrated, and often demanded attribute of modern living in Western culture. Dispositional optimism offers the bearer a general sense of resilience throughout life and an existential haven from death in advanced illness. As the patient emphatically states in line 13, "("Doctor, I'm the two percent ")", optimism can potentially appear to immunize us to evidence about what has happened to many others.

However, despite maintaining a committed, optimistic stance the patient is also "extremely bothered" by uncertainty about the future course of illness. The psychologist Leon Festinger proposes that distress can arise when one holds two opposed ideas, and that we seek to reduce this "cognitive dissonance" by changing whichever idea is easier to change at the time (Festinger 1962). In this situation, it is plausible that the patient's idea of "being the two percent" is dynamically contrasting with the equally present thought that the doctors might be right. Or, at a more fundamental level, there may be a dissonance between: "I don't want to die" and "I don't want to pursue cure-focused treatments that make me suffer." (Her stated preferences for end-of-life care favor a comfort over longevity tradeoff.)

Epidemiological analysis of participants in this study observed that optimists were at higher risk than others to experience distressing prognostic uncertainty as their awareness of nearing death grew (Gramling et al. 2017). One plausible explanation is that the belief that "I am the two percent" eventually becomes harder to maintain, leaving optimists particularly unprepared for the "sudden" awareness of death. The next conversation demonstrates one approach that we see commonly in Palliative Care settings for navigating the dissonant ideas of living and dying.

10.8 There's always gonna be some part of your brain

The following exchange involves a 85-year-old woman with stage-four ovarian cancer. She has a high school degree, no religious affiliation and is financially secure. She describes having "no idea" about whether she is likely to live for a year and is unsure about whether she would trade comfort over longevity in the last months of her life. She reports her overall quality-of-life to be a 5 out of 10 and is "quite a bit" bothered by uncertainty about what to expect from the course of her illness. The Palliative Care physician with whom she is speaking estimates her survival time as between two weeks and three months. She died 38 days after this conversation, which begins with the physician exploring whether she wishes to hear his opinion about prognosis.

1 MD: How do you feel about that,=>Some people find it helpful< and some
2   people really don't want to ↑°know°. (3.5)
3 Pt: °I'm not sure how I feel about it. ° =I'm I'm still Oh God please cure
4   me? =Uh hoping for a cure:. (1.8)

5 MD: You know I- think that's really normal. So I think (.) that (2.2) that that's
6   something that most patients that have cancer tell us is that even though
7   they've hea:rd (0.8) you know that this isn't curable that there's always
8   gonna be some part of your brain-
9 Pt: [uh]
10 MD: [That is] just (0.5) saying (0.2) you know like (0.5) you never know
11   what's gonna happen. (1.0) Um (0.5) I also have to say that (0.8) that
12   it seems like (0.5) you're doing- you know you're talking about the bills
13   and like (0.5) getting things: (.) together.=and so I think that (0.5) that
14   your actions at least speak to the fact that you're-
15 Pt: [Prepared].
16 MD: [We've heard] a lot that you're preparing (1.0) so I think that that's
17   really normal ↑to (0.5) you know to have like (0.5) the (0.5) you know
18   (.) like (.) we call it >like the medical thing< for it is hope for the best
19   and prepare for the worst=But (0.5) it seems like that's a lot of what
20   you're doing. (3.2) Um so I think as far as (1.0) would it help to talk a
21   little bit about what (0.2) what to expect going forward with this breathing
22   and the different scenarios and how we might manage it? (2.5)
23 Pt: °Well I have a feeling I should wait until they find out exactly what's
24   caus:ing it.°
25 MD: Mm-hmm,=That's true. (1.2)
26 Pt: And then talk about it. (4.8)

Similar to the preceding example, this patient demonstrates her fear of dying in line 3 when she appeals to God to cure her. Unlike the previous conversation, the Palliative Care physician normalizes the human need to hope to be cured and suggests that this hope resides in "some part of your brain," apart from the implied other part that recognizes cure is unlikely to happen. She further offers an observation that the patient has done some things that are inconsistent with expecting to live much longer, in order to "prepare." She names this "hope for the best, prepare for the worst" approach, which is commonly taught in Palliative Care training programs (Back et al. 2003). They appear to arrive at this mutual understanding that both hoping and preparing are indeed happening. However, when the physician in line 21 offers to further discuss how to prepare to control potential suffering due to her incurable shortness of breath, the patient indicates effectively that she is not ready to prepare further until she learns more news about pending diagnostic tests.

*For instances of **ambivalence toward Palliative Care**, see 2.2, 9.2, 8.5, 8.2, 8.1, 7.3. For **metaphors of hoping vs. preparing**, see 7.4, 4.4, 10.8, 6.4, 7.1, 10.10.*

10.9 A magical thing

Here, we revisit a conversation from Chapter Four, this time from a prognostic perspective. The following is a Palliative Care physician speaking with a 66-year-old woman who is Christian, holds an Associate's Degree, and is financially secure. She has stage-four lung cancer and reports her overall quality-of-life as a 3 out of 10. She is not sure about her preferences about comfort-vs.-longevity tradeoff in the focus of her treatments in the last months of her life. She is "quite a bit" bothered by prognostic uncertainty, but reports it is very likely she will live for more than a year. The physician expects her to live for 2 weeks to 3 months; she lived for 11 days after this conversation. The excerpt begins with the patient describing the task she gave to her oncologist earlier that same day:

```
1  Pt:   Nope. (1.2) That his job tonight is to go home and dream? (1.2) <He got to go
2         in his little brain≥ (0.5) make a little microtape (1.2) come out of that dream
3         (.) play that microtape >which is gonna help fix me.< ((laughter)) (0.8) It's
4         the job I gave him. (0.2)
5  MD:   You gave him a job to fix you,
6  Pt:   [Yeah.]
7  FM:   [Yeah.] (0.8)
8  FM:   °That's his job for the night.° ((laughter))
9  Pt:   Do you see where I'm that (1.2) optimisti- You know. (1.0)
10 MD:   Which is fine. (1.0) Nobody wants to (0.2) encourage you not to be
11        optimistic. (0.5) The question is: (0.5) well- (.) may I ask a direct
12        question? (0.8) What's going on with you and what does it mean. (0.2)
13        =What are the main (0.2) medical problems you're confronting right
14        now. (1.8)
15 Pt:   The breathing. (0.5)
16 MD:   Okay. (0.8) And what's the matter with it. (0.5)
17 Pt:   I can't breathe.
18 MD:   Okay. (0.8) And do you know why that is? (1.8)
19 Pt:   >Because I got tumors.<
20 PD:   Okay. (1.2) And (0.5) what are the treatments for those tumors? (0.8)
21 Pt:   There isn't any. =But there could al:ways be a magical thing.=I
22        believe. (0.8)
23 MD:   Gotcha. (0.4) Okay. (0.5) Okay.
24 Pt:   I believe that god can °do anything,°
25 MD:   Okay. (0.8) So I want to see if I get you right. =You understand that
26        (0.8) your breathing (1.0) is (.) in peril, (0.2)
```

27	Pt:	Right, (0.8)
28	MD:	>And that the <u>reason</u> for the breathing being in peril< (0.2) is (.) the
29		tumors (1.2) and there's no (.) no <u>hu</u>man (.) fixing of that. =There's
30		no treatment for that. (0.5)
31	Pt:	Yeah.
32	MD:	And you're <u>hope</u>ful you'll get <u>better</u> nonethel<u>ess.</u>
33	Pt:	<u>Right.</u>
34	MD:	>That's fair enough.< (1.5) <u>E</u>ven with the hope I want to ask (0.8)
35		what do you understand will happen if that <u>doesn't</u> happen. =If it can't
36		be fixed. (0.2) If god (0.5) doesn't (0.5) [fix <u>that</u>]
37	Pt:	[To be ho]nest with you >I'm not gonna look at it that way.> (1.5)
38	MD:	Okay.
39	Pt:	I know you might think I'm <u>weird</u> but- (0.5)
40	MD:	There's <u>noth</u>ing weird about it, =We want to talk about this in a way
41		you're <u>will</u>ing to and you want to. (1.2) The reason this matters though

The fundamental idea of "patient-centered communication" is that high-quality communication encourages physicians to see the patient's situation through both a clinical lens and from the patient's perspective (Epstein 2007). Doing so should create a health care environment where patients and physicians understand one another, even when one might believe in miracles and the other does not. Palliative Care is often consulted in situations where clinicians are worried that patients are mistakenly making decisions that are not in their best interest – such as pursuing hurtful cure-oriented therapies with little chance of success. This excerpt above begins with a quite lucid description of the patient's hopes that a cure will come to her oncologist in a dream. After the physician gently asks permission to "ask a direct question," what ensues is a relatively systematic, logical, and forthright sequence of turns in which the physician confirms that the patient is clearly aware of the medical condition's severity and the lack of further "human" solutions.

Despite the physician's rather crisp efficiency in clarifying that there are no current treatments, the undaunted patient shares her belief in "magical things" and that God can "do anything." Unlike in the example above in 10.8, the patient stops the physician from exploring with her how to prepare for "if it can't be fixed" saying, "to be honest, I'm not going to look at it that way." Nonetheless, after they share a mutual face-honoring exchange about her perspective not being "weird" and confirming that the physician wishes to "talk about this in a way that she is willing to," the physician makes one last attempt to explore important and imminent treatment choices with a volley about "the reason this matters, though..." in line 41.

10.10 Someone won't be there

Much prognostic and decision-making activity among families is shaped by very concrete questions about how their loved one will be attended to over long hours, days, and weeks of serious illness. The concern is logistical and existential at once, as demonstrated in the following conversation. The patient is identified by family proxy as a 93-year-old white woman and as financially secure, reporting high-school-level education and Christian religious affiliation. She has been diagnosed with an unknown stage-four cancer. Family members believe she is "very unlikely" to live for a year, and her clinician-rated survival prognosis at the time of the following consultation is fewer than two weeks. In fact, she lived 11 days beyond this consultation, i.e., concordant with clinical expectations. The health care proxy strongly ranks the patient's end-of-life goal as "comfort over longevity," rates her "global" quality-of-life over the previous two days at a three out of ten, and is "quite a bit" bothered by prognostic uncertainty. The clinician speaking is a Palliative Care nurse practitioner.

```
 1 NP:    Um (0.5) I mean we have to look (0.8) watch her over [the next,]
 2 FM:                                                         [Yeah.  ]
 3 NP:    Couple of days. (1.0) Um (.) but (1.2) we wouldn't be surprised if it's
 4        (0.2) like days °to ↑weeks.°
 5 FM:    Uh huh. (0.5)
 6 NP:    °So.° (1.0)
 7 FM:    Yeah I noticed she's really come down °°fast,°°
 8 NP:    Mm hmm
 9 FM:    Extremely fast,
10 NP:    Mm hmm.
11 FM:    Yeah since (1.2)
12 FM2:   S:::ince, (0.5)
13 FM:    She just (.) uh- (.) I mean once she started going down hill (.) it's just
14        been going down hill (1.0) You know. (0.2) So (1.2) you know. (0.2)
15        It's no surprise to us really. (0.8)
16 Uk:    And at ninety-three [rather than,    ]
17 FM:                        [Yeah.           ]
18 Uk:    lingering?
19 FM:    Yeah
20 Uk:    Had a good life.
21 FM:    Sh- she (.) doesn't want to be like that. =She's told us many times.=She
22        (0.2) she doesn't want to live like that. (1.2) °You know (0.5) but. °
```

23 FM2: Who <u>does</u>, ((chuckle))
24 FM: Yeah. (0.8) Yeah. (1.0)
25 FM2: °Yeah.° (0.2)

There is consensus already among family members, friends, and the Palliative Care nurse practitioner here that the patient is actively dying. And yet, the discussion of prognosis and decision-making is here only in its incipient stages, as is demonstrated in the next sequence below:

1   FM: But (.) for (0.5) how we feel about (0.5) um (.) her (0.5) as far as <u>food</u>
2   and stuff like we're just- .hhh (0.2) I mean (0.2) <she <u>can't</u> reach a call
3   button if she (0.2) if she needs to.> .hh (0.2) And she <u>can't</u>: feed herself
4   at a:ll and she <u>can't</u>: bring a <u>cup</u> to her <u>so</u>: .hh (0.5) um (0.8) you know
5   we were just (0.5) kind of nervous cause her <u>food</u> was still there (0.5)
6   and (.) not that (.) >we don't know if anybody came in and tried to <u>do</u>
7   anything< but um (0.5) she had some of the <u>orange</u> ice and _____ had
8   brought her some <u>apple</u>sauce and she did take a little bit of <u>that</u>. (0.5) But
9   um (1.0) um (.) those few things (.) that (0.2) that was a little bit what
10   we're nervous about (0.2) you know? (.) that somebody won't be <u>there</u>.
11   (0.5) She can't (.) she won't eat any foods like the foods that (0.5) are
12   there on her <u>plate</u>. (0.5) You know. =she's (1.0) she's not like <u>that</u>,

What matters most to the family members here is that the patient not suffer neglect or absence in the hospital, and that they will be able to rest assured that she will continue to be comfortable and accompanied. This is not only a worry, but also a decision-making topic, to the extent that they must individually consider how to formulate their visiting and care-taking schedules in line with a comfort-only treatment plan.

For family member's **concerns about food and feeding,** *see 3.6, 8.4. For* **speculations about other absent clinicians,** *see 7.5, 2.2, 2.3, 7.6, 9.5, 8.5, 7.1, 4.2, 7.2.*

10.11 I'm just waiting for it to happen

Often, patients with long-term serious illness are very familiar with the prospect of dying and express stances toward it that range from the practical to the stoic. The patient in the following conversation self-identifies as a 54-year-old white man and as financially secure, reporting Associate's-level education and Christian religious affiliation. He has been diagnosed with a stage-four colon cancer. He believes he is unable to estimate his prognosis and is only slightly bothered by prognostic uncertainty, while his clinician-rated survival prognosis at the time of the following consultation is three to six months. In fact, he lived eight days beyond this consultation, i.e., drastically shorter than clinically expected. The patient strongly ranks his end-of-life goals as "comfort over longevity," and he rates his "global" quality-of-life over the previous two days – i.e., physical, emotional, social, spiritual, and financial quality – at an eight out of ten. The following portion of talk occurred during the first visit of the Palliative Care team, represented here by a nurse practitioner.

1	Pt:	>It's kind of <u>hard</u> if you don't have a lot of information< so. -
2	NP:	So if (0.2) um so it sounds <u>like</u> if ah chemotherapy were an option is
3		<u>that</u> what you would want to try?
4	Pt:	I would take it again
5		[if- if it]
6	NP:	[Okay.]
7	Pt:	Was an <u>op</u>tion.
8	NP:	Okay (0.2) And- <u>and</u> (0.2) just to (.) you know explain a little <u>bit</u> more
9		about hos↑pice (0.5) um so if (.) <u>if</u> hospice were and Dr. _____ a:ll feel
10		that (0.5) unfortunately this disease is not able to be turned around-
11	Pt:	Yeah he <u>told</u> me that already so [um]
12	NP:	[Then -]
13	Pt:	[Well <u>that's</u> what I'm saying]
14	NP:	[and would you]
15	Pt:	If- If worse came to worse I <u>would</u> go to hospice.
16	NP:	Okay.
17	Pt:	I would rather be in <u>hos</u>pice than ( ) (0.5) >I don't want to go to somebody's
18		<<u>house</u> and (.) °have them come home and find me°
19	NP:	Right, (1.0) So-
20	Pt:	Or b:leed out on ↑their- (0.8) I just .hhhhhh the- the woman I I I <u>liked</u> the
21		woman I lived with sh: (.) I've known her for like 30 ↑years.
22	NP:	Uh huh.
23	Pt:	But um. (0.8) >I just don't want °her to come home< and have me uh -°
24	NP:	Yeah.
25	Pt:	She lives like seven miles out of _____ on the <u>woo:</u>ds (1.0) And it's like
26		<u>no</u> I don't want to do ↑that you <u>know</u> (1.0) I just don't want to end up.=I
27		mean even if it- if it happens °it happens I've ↑decided.° (1.0)
28	NP:	Yeah.
29	Pt:	I've been <u>here</u> I'm just °waiting for it to ↑<u>happen</u>.° (1.2)

For this patient, the necessary decisions are those that diminish the likelihood that he will die in a way or in a setting that will bring difficulty to others, and yet he is uncertain how he can take precautions to make sure that such circumstances are avoided. Overall, he expresses the sense that he is merely "waiting for death" to come and that there is little decision-making left for him to undertake.

For patients' **imaginings about death**, see 3.2, 10.1, 4.3, 8.4, 3.6. For **patients' concerns about becoming a burden**, see 8.3. For expressions of **waiting for death**, see 2.5.

10.12 You wouldn't leave the bed

We are interested in situations in which a clinician issues a rather predictive, prescriptive expectation of what is to come, even if it is not a direct description of disease progression (on directives, see Craven and Potter 2010). In this case, the prediction is about how restricted a patient's mobility will be at home, once he leaves the hospital into hospice care. The patient in the following conversation self-identifies as an 80-year-old white man and as financially secure, reporting graduate level education and no religious affiliation. He has been diagnosed with a stage-four cancer, but it has not been biopsied. He believes he is "very unlikely" to live for a year and is moderately bothered by prognostic uncertainty, while his clinician-rated survival prognosis is two weeks to three months. In fact, he continued to live for 34 days after this interview, which means that both his and the clinicians' prognosis estimate were accurate. He ranks his end-of-life goals as "comfort over longevity," and he rates his "global" quality-of-life over the previous two days – physical, emotional, social, spiritual, and financial – at a zero out of ten. The following portion of talk occurred during the first visit of the Palliative Care team, close to the beginning of the conversation. The clinician speaking is a Palliative Care physician.

1 MD: I think (0.5) especially if we're looking at (.) <u>home</u> (0.5) rea<u>lis</u>tically you
2   probably would not leave. (.) the hospital bed (0.8)
3 Pt: Would not leave the hospital bed.
4 MD: <u>You</u> would not leave the bed.
5 Pt: [Yes.]
6 MD: [Except] for: (0.2) <u>very</u> rare occasions where you might (0.5) go in a
7   wheelchair,
8 Pt: Which takes (0.5) <u>falling</u> risk down to <u>nothing</u>?
9 Sp: °Mm-hmm.°

10 MD: Right. Um and takes the toilet issue,
11 Dt: Right. [Mm-hmm.]
12 MD: [off   ]
13 Pt: Take that off the <u>table.</u>
14 Dt: Yep.
15 MD: Yeah. >So it would be using bedpans<I think (0.2) just from you know
16   the way you described, and what (0.2) °I was reading in the chart° (0.2)
17   with where you <u>are</u> in terms of your <u>strength,</u> (0.5) <u>I</u> don't think >you're
18   going to get out of the bed much,<
19 Pt: Right?
20 MD: If at all.
21 Pt: Right. I ag<u>ree.</u>
22 MD: Um.
23 Dt: So how many how much services can we get <u>in:to</u>: (.) the house? (0.5)
24 MD: Most- uh huh. =if we're talking about the <u>hos</u>pice >provided services<
25 Dt: Yeah.
26 MD: >It's about< (0.5) they <u>say</u> a couple hours.
27 Sp: °Mm-hmm.°
28 MD: I think <u>five</u> to seven days a week depending?

We see in line 3–4 that the physician makes a direct, unqualified, on-record prediction about the patient's near-term restricted mobility. The sentence "You wouldn't leave the bed" doubles as a description and a directive, by which he both characterizes and prescribes a course of conduct for the patient at home. What we find interesting is that this sort of direct prediction is taken up unflinchingly by the family, who appear to find the certainty of the physician's stance on this question reassuring. Later in the conversation, the physician counteracts the face-threat issued with a gesture of options and magnanimity in lines 12–14 below. The current topic is outpatient hospice services:

1 MD: <u>Each</u> one of those actually has their own: (0.5) <u>separate cen</u>ter? (0.2) that's
2   kind of like a mini: <u>hos</u>pital? (.) for hospice and for com↑fort. =And so
3   most of the time if <u>that's,</u> what's needed=you go there.
4 Dt: Oh.
5 MD: So if <u>things</u> start to go out of con↑trol ((coughing)) you're not- you have
6   that <u>whole</u> (.) <u>back-up.</u>
7 Dt: You <u>go</u> there.=you don't go to the hospital.=you go there?
8 MD: Sometimes you come to the <u>hos</u>pital.
9 Dt: Mm-hmm.

10 MD: >It depends upon the beds and everything.=Or if you want to come back
11   here< we've- we've had >patients who come back here< and (.) that's
12   because they <u>prefer</u> (0.2) and we're welcome to °have you° (0.5) Wherever
13   you prefer to go.=But I mean there's (1.0) there's a lot of: (0.5) plans B C D
14   that- that kind of get built (.) in the- background (0.5) just in case we need
15   them.
16 Dt: °Mm-hmm.°

The physician's unequivocal directive about the nature of the patient's future
mobility is tempered in the sequence above by a welcoming reminder that there
are always multiple options available for augmenting the care that the patient is
receiving at home.

For instances of **frankness and indirection**, see 2.1, 4.5, 6.1–2, 7.3, 8.3, 8.5, 9.2.
For discussions about **going home**, see 4.1, 4.5, 5.4. For discussions about **options**
for end-of-life care scenarios, see 3.1, 3.2, 3.5, 4.2, 5.5.

10.13 Insights and implications from Chapter 10

As prognosis and prognostication are among the most discussed and measured
components of Palliative Care communication thus far in US-based research,
we have decided to close this book with a review of a number of conversations
that appeared in previous chapters, in which prognosis was one of the primary
projects. Though prognosis has been a major focus of recent study in Palliative
Care, addressing a century of aversion to prognosis talk in US medicine, prognosis is no straightforward procedure. It involves complex balancing of interactional, subjective, intersubjective, physiological, ethical, and logistical
questions about the future. We hope to have shown in this chapter a range of
scenarios in which prognostic communication arises and what effects it tends
to have on the overall arc of communication. As discussed in the introduction
to this chapter, prognosis is a practice and a communicative genre that has
fallen out of general medical training since the 1870s, and it most frequently
falls to the young discipline of Palliative Care to fill the historical and discursive gap left. Studying how, when, and for what purposes patients and clinicians talk meaningfully about prognosis will require ongoing interactional
research.

11 Concluding remarks

Your social situation is not your country cousin.
— Erving Goffman, "The Neglected Situation" (1964: 134)

"Something important has been neglected," wrote the Canadian-American sociologist Erving Goffman ominously, in a brief essay now more than fifty years ago. Though "Each year new social determinants of speech behavior are reported," (Goffman 1964: 133), these prospective features of communication analysis, which Goffman saw researchers eagerly introducing in the 1960s, were often put forth in isolation rather than in a holistic relation. There was good reason for this: how can one operationalize holism, anyway? How can any discrete component of linguistic practice matter, if it is just one among many moving, messy parts, local in its specificity and tragically difficult to reproduce? Driven by an optimistic vision of what could ultimately be learned regarding humans in conversation with one another, researchers of Goffman's era put forth more and more tools, angles, and components by which to analytically disambiguate this most central of human activities. But, so Goffman claimed, the "situation" remained somehow still neglected.

In his time, Goffman did not quite think that situations of spoken interaction were being neglected whole by researchers, but that they were being left under-complicated, or that the implications of situatedness were treated as an afterthought. Models of power and distance that portrayed the social and institutional context of speaking as dry equations rather than as soaked and transformative realities made him hunger for a mode of analysis that regarded the speech situation as one of "mutual monitoring possibilities" (135), where such social dynamics as power and politeness are being recognized, negotiated, undermined, and reinforced by all participants in every moment of the interaction.

Studies of communication in Palliative Care settings can only benefit from Goffman's reminder that "what is going on" (1974: 46) in the space of interaction is not just the sum of component analytic ingredients. Since the threshold moment of Temel et al. (2011) and its consequences for hospital policy, attempts to determine the "measurable" elements of Palliative Care as a clinical and billable specialty have been putting pressure on the discipline to produce a de-situated, reproducible, ingredients-based vision of the Palliative Care consultation. This is reasonable, to the extent that it is reasonable to clamor for models that work and deliver good results. But oftentimes the analytic means by which we may attempt to render these elements visible obscure more about the realities of patient-clinician-family interactions than they capture.

https://doi.org/10.1515/9781501504570-011

In *Palliative Care Conversations,* we have attempted to show that patients and families tell us a different story, one represented at length and in context in the nine foregoing chapters. Let us review briefly the situated elements emerging from this composite story, which may guide not only future research but also policy-making and teaching within Palliative Care and related fields. The following are not discrete ingredients, but dynamic discursive and interactional features frequently encountered in the Palliative Care consultation–as its "table is set" by patients, family members, other specialists, social and political ideology at large, and indeed Palliative Care clinicians themselves.

1.   Patients are active, expert, and competent social and institutional analysts.
"I listen very carefully to words," says a 56-year-old patient with stage-four cervical cancer, cited in our introduction. She is saying this not merely to describe her own character or to introduce herself, but also to put her clinical team on notice that their granular linguistic practices – particular metaphors, turns of phrase, implicatures – matter to her.

2.   Patients and families suffering long-term serious illness often take on genres of institutional hospital talk – as a combination of strategy, accommodation, expertise, and habit.
Even such minor details as saying "I'm the wife" as opposed perhaps to "I'm his wife" (2.1) are indicative of an apparent assimilation to ways of speaking that presume the need for a shared expedient code for the Palliative Care consultation, i.e., taking on the presumed perspective of the clinical team.

3.   Palliative Care clinicians appear to be at their most effective when not beginning the consultation with conventional patient-centered volleys.
The clinician in 2.1 begins the consultation with a rather clinician-centered description of the discipline of Palliative Care, speaking about "what I typically get asked to do here in the hospital." This approach, in turn, helps model for patients and families exactly what range of services he can provide. It takes the onus off of them, at least in the beginning of the consultation, to self-represent or to conjure *ex nihilo* an idea about what this strange and sometimes foreboding new discipline of Palliative medicine can offer them in that moment, particularly given the fact that seriously-ill hospitalized persons are often exhausted from repeating their histories to ever-new personnel.

4.   Patients and families use a range of their own vernacular speech genres – business, the outdoors, etc. – to frame their own serious illnesses. Clinicians can effectively take up these cues and genres for interactional benefit to all.

It is not necessarily the case that a patient is avoiding talking about death when he/she frames a health situation in terms that appear less than adequately existential in the moment. Particularly the patient in conversation 4.1 deliberately fends off discourse genres that he deems inappropriate for his situation, by announcing, about him and his family, that "We're not deep thinkers."

5. **Palliative Care is a symbolically overdetermined specialty, and patients/families usually have some pre-formed, skeptical notions about what it means.**
In conversation 3.1, the patient is attempting to politely 'size up' the Palliative Care service personnel, as if they were a valiant but opposing team. "How many people are in Palliative Care?" he asks – simultaneously querying their legitimacy as a potential aid to him and as a potential menace. The remainder of the interaction is thus decisive in how such symbolic overdeterminations, emanating from broader media and political discourses, but also from the marked absence of prognosis discourse in other specialties, are either reinforced or revised.

6. **Clinicians in Palliative Care consultations tend to use hedging and indirection as resources, while patients often see fit to dispense early with "beating around the bush".**
"It's obviously terminal," says one 80-year-old patient when the physician asks him "What is your understanding of kind of where things are with your disease or what's going on" (2.1). In 2.2, the patient appears to be attempting to triage multiple different institutional priorities and wants the clinician to get to the point as quickly as possible.

7. **Dying in hospital is an experience shaded by multiply overlayered historical discourses.**
In conversation 6.2, the patient is using the term "mercy killing" to reflect on her own perceived role in her father's death in a context of life-limiting illness, decades ago. Now in a similar situation as her father appears to have been, the patient transfers the discursive framework of "mercy killing" and its conceptual tools from her father's generation to her own. Thus, Palliative Care interactions need to be cautious about the fallacy of presentism – i.e., the notion that the discourses of today are the most active, influential, or meaningful for patients in conceptualizing their own experiences of dying.

8. **Descriptive introductions of the field of Palliative Care should be keyed to practical needs and results and should err on the side of explicit enumeration, wide applicability, and added benefits.**
The clinician in conversation 2.5 exemplifies an approach that highlights the demonstrated track record, the broad popular appeal, and the somewhat luxurious

benefits of Palliative Care service (including Reiki therapy, massage, pets and music therapy, etc.). Though this may appear to be a form of Public Relations management, it is an effective way for families to reframe Palliative Care as a value-added service, rather than one that signals imminent death or deficits in curability.

9. Unexpected frankness is often a useful tool in Palliative Care settings.
The clinician in conversation 5.1 contradicts the patient curt response about their well-being ("I'm fine") with the on-record face-threat "No you're not." This turns out to be an effective rapport-building tool, precisely because Palliative Care is so structurally and discursively unlike other hospital-based medical specialties.

10. Psychological conceptions of denial or dissonance are often inadequate categories for understanding patients' choices not to pursue comfort measures.
In conversation 4.4, even after clinicians have made several explicit prognostic volleys, the patient announces to the clinical team that she has reasonably decided to not to entertain 'worst case scenarios.' Her stance is something fundamentally different than denial, in that she has surveyed all evidence given her and decided it is the most reasonable course of action in her situation to rely on divine salvation as her best resource for pragmatism and proper planning.

Of course, each of the dynamics listed and exemplified above are webs of practice that emerge not only in local hospital landscapes, but from within broader socio-political debates about death and dying. One Palliative Care patient in the current study tapped into this macro-political matrix directly, reporting to her Palliative Care physician during an initial consultation that: "I just don't want to be Terri Schiavo." Despite the unequivocal frankness of this request, she did not go on to specify whether her negative association with Schiavo meant that she did not want (a) to be kept alive indefinitely in a comatose or vegetative state, (b) to have her end-of-life decisions made by government officials, (c) to have her private affairs discussed in the international media and talk-show circuit, (d) to be the object of a rancorous family dispute, (e) to have her illness serve as a test-case for party platforms or case law, or (f) to be remembered primarily for the portion of her life she spent unconscious, rather than for her activities and identity prior to serious illness. Nonetheless, all of these potential implicatures together animate her remark about Terri Schiavo, who had died in hospice in March 2005, ten years prior to the patient's own hospitalization (Neporent 2015). Though Ms. Schiavo had never engaged Palliative Care services over the course of her 15-year hospitalization, this person's ambiguous reference to her ten years later in our study is, in some senses, typical of both the multi-layered idiom and the discursive polycentricity of Palliative Care decision-making conversations.

11.1 From 'Death Panels' to *Dying in America*

At the American Heartland Forum in Columbia, Missouri/USA, on 3 February 2012, then Presidential candidate, Sen. Rick Santorum (R-PA), gave a stump speech in which he rekindled the "death panel" rancor of 2009, claiming that "Elderly people in the Netherlands don't go to the hospital. They go to another country because they're afraid because of budget purposes they won't come out of that hospital" (Williamson 2012). Leveraging the apocryphal Dutch 'Do Not Euthanize Me" bracelets in service of an anti-Affordable Care Act plank, the candidate vividly linked socialized medicine to systematic, mass euthanasia in "old Europe's" hospitals.

This electoral and legislative tenor put several health care fields, including Palliative Care, in a tough spot nationally. In an attempt to "bridge the spectrum of the health care debate," the Institutes of Medicine released a 515-page report in 2014 called *Dying in America*, compiled by a committee of doctors, nurses, public health officials, and business people. The *Dying in America* report cited statistical evidence that, in 2009, 23% of US residents believed the Affordable Care Act allowed clinicians to make decisions about whether a patient would be allowed to die or not and – more importantly – that 36% were unsure. National professional organizations such as the Center to Advance Palliative Care were aware of these statistics and the complex ambivalence they represented. It was clear that Palliative Care clinicians and their institutional advocates needed simultaneously to combat deliberate politicization, raise public awareness about their clinical purpose, ensure accurate representation of their work in public discussions as well as internally in their institutional settings, and – all the while – continue to provide the care they were certified and trained to offer. These multiple, simultaneous tasks coalesced in a new push for training initiatives, research programs, and talking-point templates for discussing what Palliative Care is and is not. The phrase "an extra layer of support" became a common short-hand for explaining to patients and families in the midst of serious illness what Palliative Care's specific contribution was to the clinical landscape of the hospital. But this and similar phrases introduced their own set of pragmatic ambiguities.

While the authoritative industry report *Dying in America* insisted that communication and conversation were key to improving patients' access to a dignified death in hospital settings, the report offered few guidelines for how to model, reflect, or analyze situated patient-clinician dialogue. Indeed, very little was reported in *Dying in America* about actual linguistic or conversational behaviors, or about how to improve them in practical settings. Cast as an urgent, broad objective, 'better communication' remained an ethical ideal to strive for, despite a simultaneous trend in hospital billing and auditing protocols that discouraged time-intensive clinical conversation between physicians and patients.

11.2 Constitutional questions: Speech, action, and hastening death

In its undetailed urgency around communication and conversation, the *Dying in America* report was a reflection of – as much as a reflection on – twenty years of end-of-life care discussions in the age of patient-centered medicine. Language-in-use had always been, in some senses, the undertheorized and under analyzed elephant in the room. In 1997, the US Supreme Court had decided unanimously that the State of New York could intervene to prevent a physician from allowing a patient to choose comfort-only medical care. Though the decision in this case, called Vacco v. Quill (521 US 793), was issued as "unanimous," the Justices of the Rehnquist Court handed down six distinct opinions (one majority, five concurring), indicating that the unanimity of the verdict was far from univocal. In case-law and constitutional terms, at issue in the case was whether the 14th Amendment to the US Constitution, and specifically its "equal protection clause", could be interpreted as recognizing a fundamental right to die.

More specifically, Chief Justice Rehnquist's written opinion took recourse to the legal principle of intent, dividing physician agency into two categories, which in their formulation are strikingly beholden to semantic and grammatical parsing. When a physician respects a person's wishes to die, wrote Rehnquist, she does not necessarily *intend* the patient to die. In contrast, administering any form of assistance in the act of dying is tantamount to intentional killing, which was in violation of New York State law. According to Rehnquist, the 14th Amendment protects a person's right to die, but not to have their death facilitated. In the absence of clinical or sociolinguistic data to support and situate the distinction, "letting die" vs. "hastening death" were ruled to be sturdy empirical categories, immanent in the Constitution.

From the outset, then, the formative Vacco v. Quill precedent banning the 'hastening of death' was achieved not through analysis of actual physician-patient-family dialogue and deliberation, but through an idealist and legalist tableau of active vs. passive agency, a distinction to which very little actual clinical or otherwise intersubjective activity corresponds, as we see in the conversations throughout this book. Conversation – the detailed internal workings of which were all but ignored in the deliberations – became with this ruling a statutory territory that was to be regulated in grammatical terms encased in a positivistic logic about intent. The Rehnquist Court's reliance on strong, extralinguistic characterizations of decision-making activity in conversation has since 1997 constituted a lasting subtext for Palliative Care conversations.

As Palliative Care prepares for its next quarter-century of practical inquiry into the most effective, just, and compassionate forms of interaction that might emerge in hospital-based communication with seriously-ill people, the field will need to continue to bear in mind the intersectional, symbolic, and social nature of these interactions. Not only are patients and families negotiating the immediate spatial sociology of their clinical floor, the sometimes-opaque logic of 'rounding' and referring according to which clinical interactions emerge, and the processes and procedures of a large bureaucratic institution, they are also negotiating freighted, chronodiverse, and complex moral and social discourses about dying in our societies. Approaches to communication that atomize ingredients of conversation will tend to lack the ability to bridge these spheres and to link them to other complex symbolic systems such as family, kinship, finances, spiritual practice, and affect. We believe that taking to heart individual cases of interaction, in their most granular detail, can help clinicians and policy-makers arrive at customs, policies, and modes that most adequately apprehend the stated needs of patients. We consider the participants in this study, therefore, to be our primary teachers – helping the clinical specialty of Palliative Care to learn and listen carefully to what their experiences have taught them.

11.3 Thematic questions for further inquiry

Note: In each case, the number of the subchapter exploring each respective question is given.

Morality, ethics, worldview

What kinds of moral, existential, and family-historical questions do patients pose to Palliative Care specialists, and what experiences prompt them to do so? How do Palliative Care practitioners formulate answers to such questions that, even when they are topically not "about" the patient's disease, can nonetheless play an important role in improving that patient's current quality-of-life, wholeness, and comfort? (3.2)

Social, political, and personal history

How do Palliative Care clinicians address historical discourses like "mercy killing", when these themes and idioms are raised by patients? (3.2)

How can past experiences be best engaged as a resource for current clinical, social, spiritual, and interactional needs? (3.2)

Should clinicians be expected to assimilate all of the various aspects of a seriously-ill person's medical history before speaking with the patient? (9.1)

Is speaking with a seriously-ill person without being able to account for all aspects of the medical history bound for rapport loss? (9.1)

Speech genres and cultural repertoires

Are there ways of speaking and interactional resources that family members take up, which are simply unavailable to clinicians? (3.5)

What does it sound like when a clinician does not have access to the repertoire or experience necessary to build rapport with a patient? (5.2)

How do patients, clinicians, and family members knowingly or unknowingly use cultural and media references that create barriers for communication? (5.2)

How do additional-language speakers of English harness the complex ideological resources of English, and particularly of US American English, to characterize themselves and their needs vis-à-vis health-care discourses? (6.4)

How do patients "unlock" the codes of clinical discourse in ways that yield critical insight and practical benefit to them? (6.5)

What kinds of clinician-initiated metaphors about illness and survival tend to be quite well received by patients suffering serious illness? (9.4)

Physiological constraints on speech and expression

How do patients using an assistive technology to speak achieve a holistic or meaningful presentation of self in Palliative Care settings? (4.5)

What features emerge in part by virtue of the stylistic constraint of the speech-generating device? What unique stylistic power inheres in these contributions, which may not be able to come forth in other forms of unconstrained speech in interaction? (6.1)

Humor, rapport, and irony

How do irony, disabusal, and divestment from conventional approaches to rapport often constitute the basis of rapport within Palliative Care settings? (5.1)

What kinds of cultural and media references can help promote rapport? (5.2)

How do conversations that draw on irony and dark humor help establish a collective epistemic stance through which patients and clinicians co-construct their deliberations? (5.4)

What level of humor is appropriate for various participants in Palliative Care consultations? (9.4)

Politeness, honor, and respect

When do patients and families find "dispensing with the niceties" to be a relief, as they seek to come to terms with the complicated questions that await? (5.1)

What sorts of resources and rituals do clinicians invoke to honor the patient as an active participant in his/her treatment and as an autonomous being independent of his/her illness? (5.5)

How do patients tend to characterize and illustrate the complex humanity of other clinicians they work with? How do Palliative Care clinicians respond to, or participate in, such characterizations? What kind of symbolic work gets done through these joint characterizations of the complex humanity of absent clinicians? (7.2)

Palliative Care's relationships with other disciplines

How do Palliative Care clinicians implicitly value the contributions of absent clinicians from other disciplines, when those clinicians' stances are portrayed by patients themselves? (7.1)

What symbolic work gets done in interaction when absent clinicians are invoked through reported speech or summaries of those clinicians' stances? (7.1)

Solidarity, autonomy, and representation

How and why do patients choose to be spoken for by others? (7.4)

How do surrogates describe and understand this responsibility to speak for a patient? (7.4)

How do Palliative Care clinicians respond to this division of communicative labor between patients and surrogates? (7.4)

Introductions, presentations, and responses

Is the presentation of Palliative Care tailored to the clinical situation of the patient, or does the clinician present a broader picture of the specialty and then perhaps move on to elucidate its applicability to the particular patient's situation? (2.1)

What function and value do family-initiated tellings about Palliative Care (its functions, philosophy, benefits, etc.) offer that clinician-initiated presentations may not? (3.5)

How do these conversational designs – practiced, spontaneous, or unintended as they may appear to be – elicit certain responses from patients and families, and why do they appear to do so? (2.1)

How do patients and families, as yet unfamiliar with Palliative Care as a branch of medicine, test and probe it in various ways that are not directly informational?

Are such testing-and-probing projects on the part of patients ritualistic and phatic (i.e., designed for establishing contact or "small talk"), or do they appear to have broader interactional and ideological implications? (3.1)

Power, authority, and expertise

When is the topic of "guiding the conversation" made explicit in Palliative Care conversations? (8.1)

At which junctures does such metadiscursive recourse to "guiding the conversation" seem most potentially important or, conversely, most potentially disruptive? (8.1)

What appear to be the advantages and disadvantages (to patients and clinicians) of open-ended, free-form discussion centered on "what you want to talk about," as contrasted with explicit attempts to "guide the conversation"? (8.2)

Is it of benefit for patients and families when the clinician humbles herself and describes her own fallibility? (9.5)

How can a clinician's willingness to be corrected by patients or family members be expressed early on in a consultation? (9.5)

Interactional discord, resistance, and repair

What are the techniques and premises by which patients (implicitly or explicitly) resist interaction with a Palliative Care clinician, and what preexisting and emerging circumstances prompt them to do so? (2.2)

How do phenomena of discordance in Palliative Care conversations intersect with gendered, religious, and racialized features of interaction? (2.2)

What pre-existing circumstances foment antagonism and discord in Palliative Care conversations? (5.3)

What interactional features in Palliative Care conversations exacerbate pre-existing circumstances of antagonism? (5.3)

What interactional features in Palliative Care conversations help to mitigate pre-existing circumstances of antagonism? (5.3)

How does a Palliative Care clinician come across, when persisting in her attempts to repair, or salvage, the occasion to re-present Palliative Care when met with resistance and refusal? (2.2)

How do family members express doubt or frustration with a clinician's apparent unfamiliarity with the details of a patient's health history? When such confrontations occur, how can clinicians best respond? (9.3)

Timing, logistics, and information management

What happens when family members and patients attempt to elicit specific information from Palliative Care clinicians that is beyond the scope of their roles as they've presented them? (2.2)

Under what circumstances may it be imprudent to initiate or continue a consultation? (2.2)

What items tend to be foremost in family members' minds about the nuts-and-bolts of Palliative Care, but are often not quite made clear to them in "re-presenting Palliative Care" volleys? (3.6)

Should a Palliative Care consultation be timed in specific relation to when other clinical specialties round? Is this a logistical possibility? (9.2)

When coordination of information among the involved specialist is not possible, what expectations among patients and families tend to be thwarted, and how is this expressed? (9.2)

Accommodation and interpretive literacy

How do clinicians seek to "translate" official or semi-official definitions of Palliative Care into terms they feel, spontaneously or otherwise, better fit the needs of the clinical setting? (2.4)

What kinds of interpretive practices do patients develop to discern the stances of their clinicians of various specialties? (7.3)

How might we characterize the overall literacy of discernment that patients develop through their multiple and continuous interactions with clinical personnel? (7.3)

Silence or non-communication

How and when do patients and family members forgo disclosure of their previous experiences with Palliative Care? What interactional features prompt them to do so? (3.3)

Does the Palliative Care consultation genre tend to elicit certain responses and self-characterizations as to patients' and families' *general* inclinations towards reflective talking and thinking? (4.1)

How do patients and clinicians actively collaborate in producing internally acceptable ways of speaking (and not speaking) about certain topics? How does this interactional production of discursive perimeters differ, say, from merely designating proscribed or "taboo" topics? (6.3)

References

Abbot, Andrew. 1988. *The system of the professions: An essay on the division of expert labor*. Chicago: University of Chicago Press.

Abbot, Katherine, Joni Sago, Catherine Green, Amy Abernethy and James Tulsky. 2001. Families looking back. One year after discussion of withdrawal or withholding of life sustaining support. *Critical Care Medicine* 29. 197–201.

Agar, Michael. 1996 [1980]. *The professional stranger. An informal introduction to ethnography*. 2nd edn. New York: Academic Press.

Aikhenvald, Aleksandra. Y. 2004. *Evidentiality*. Oxford: Oxford University Press.

Ajzen, Icek. 1991. The theory of planned behavior. *Organizational Behavior and Human Decision Processes* 50(2). 179–211.

Aldridge, Matthew and Ellen Barton. 2007. Establishing terminal status in end-of-life discussions. *Qualtiative Health Research* 17. 908–918.

Alexander, Stewart C., Susan Ladwig, Sally A. Norton, David J. Gramling, J. Kelly Davis, Maureen Metzger, Jane DeLuca and Robert Gramling. 2014. Emotional distress and compassionate responses in Palliative Care decision-making consultations. *Journal of Palliative Medicine* 7(5). 579–584.

Alexander, Stewart C., David K. Garner, Matthew Somoroff, David J. Gramling, Sally A. Norton and Robert Gramling. 2015. Using music[al] knowledge to represent expressions of emotions. *Patient Education and Counseling*. 98(11). 1339–1345.

Anderson, Stephen R. and Edward L. Keenan. 1985. Deixis. In Timothy Shopen (ed.), *Language typology and syntactic description*, 259–308. Cambridge: Cambridge University Press.

Angus, Derek, Amber Bonato, Walter Linde-Zwirble, Lisa Weissfeld, Scott Watson, Tim Rickert and Gordon Rubenfeld. 2004. Use of intensive care at the end of life in the United States: an epidemiologic study. *Critical Care Medicine* 32. 638–643.

Antaki, Charles. 1994. *Explaining and arguing: The social organization of accounts*. London: Sage.

Antaki, Charles. 2004. Reading minds or dealing with interactional implications? *Theory and Psychology* 14(5). 667–683.

Antaki, Charles (ed.). 2011a. *Applied conversation analysis: Intervention and change in institutional talk*. Basingstoke: Palgrave Macmillan.

Antaki, Charles. 2011b. Six kinds of applied conversation analysis. In Charles Antaki (ed.), *Applied conversation analysis: Intervention and change in institutional talk*, 1–14. Basingstoke: Palgrave Macmillan.

Antaki, Charles, Hanneke Houtkoop-Steenstra and Mark Rapley. 2000. "Brilliant. Next question...": High-grade assessment sequences in the completion of interactional units. *Research on Language and Social Interaction* 33(3). 235–262.

Antaki, Charles and Mark Rapley. 1996. 'Quality-of-life' talk: The liberal paradox of psychological testing. *Discourse & Society* 7(3). 293–316.

Ariss, Steven M. 2009. Asymmetrical knowledge claims in general practice consultations with frequently attending patients: Limitations and opportunities for patient participation. *Social Science and Medicine* 69(6). 908–919.

Appleton, Lynda and Maria Flynn. 2014. Searching for the new normal: Exploring the role of language and metaphors in becoming a cancer survivor. *European Journal of Oncology Nursing* 18. 378–384.

https://doi.org/10.1515/9781501504570-012

Atkinson, J. Maxwell. 1982. Understanding formality: Notes on the categorisation and production of 'formal' interaction. *British Journal of Sociology* 33. 86–117.

Atkinson, J. Maxwell and John Heritage (eds.,) 1984. *Structures of social action: studies in conversation analysis*. Cambridge: Cambridge University Press.

Atkinson, Paul. 1995. *Medical talk and medical work: The liturgy of the clinic*. London: Sage.

Auer, Peter. 1996. On the prosody and syntax of turn-continuations. In Elizabeth Couper-Kuhlen and Margret Selting (eds.), *Prosody in conversation: Interactional studies*, 7–100. Cambridge: Cambridge University Press.

Auer, Peter, Elizabeth Couper-Kuhlen and Frank Müller. 1999. *Language in time: The rhythm and tempo of spoken interaction*. Oxford: Oxford University Press.

Austin, John L. 1962. *How to do things with words*. Oxford: Clarendon Press.

Austin, John. L. 1970a. Performative utterances. In John L. Austin, James O. Urmson and Geoffrey J. Warnock (eds.), *Philosophical papers*, 2nd edn., 233–222. London: Oxford University Press.

Austin, John L. 1970b. *Philosophical papers*. London: Oxford University Press.

Australian Commission on Safety and Quality in Health Care. 2013. *Safety and quality of end-of-life care in acute hospitals: A background paper*. Sydney, New South Wales, Australia.

Australian Medical Association. 2014. *Position statement on end of life care and advance care planning*. Barton, ACT.

Azoulay, Élie, Frédéric Pochard, Sylvie Chevret, Charles Arich, François Brivet, Frédéric Brun, Pierre-Emmanuel Charles, Thibaut Desmettre, Didier Dubois, Richard Galliot, Maite Garrouste-Orgeas, Dany Goldgran-Toledano, Patrick Herbecq, Luc-Marie Joly, Mercé Jourdain, Michel Kaidomar, Alain Lepape, Nicolas Letellier, Olivier Marie, Bernard Page, Antoine Parrot, Pierre-Andre Radie-Talbere, Alain Sermet, Alain Tenaillon, Marie Thuong, Patrick Tulasne, Jean-Roger Le Gall, Benoît Schlemmer, the French Famirea Group. 2003. Family participation in care to the critically ill: opinions of families and staff. *Intensive Care Medicine* 29(9). 1498–1504.

Azoulay, Élie, Sylvie Chevret, Ghislaine Leleu, Frédéric Pochard, Michel Baboteu, Christophe Andre, Pierre Canoui, Jean-Roger Le Gall, Benoît Schlemmer et al. 2000. Half the families of intensive care unit patients experience inadequate communication with physicians. *Critical Care Medicine* 28. 3044–3049.

Back, Anthony, Robert M. Arnold, and Timothy E. Quill. 2003. Hope for the best, and prepare for the worst. *Annals of Internal Medicine* 138(5). 439–343.

Back, Anthony, Susan Bauer-Wu, Cynda Rushton and Joan Halifax. 2009. Compassionate silence in the patient-clinician encounter: a contemplative approach. *Journal of Palliative Medicine* 12(12). 1113–1117.

Ball, Martin J. and John K. Local. 1996. Current develpments in transcription. In Martin J. Ball and Martin Duckworth (eds.), *Advances in clinical phonetics*, 51–89. Amsterdam: John Benjamins.

Bartels, Josef, Rachel Rodenbach, Katherine Ciesinski, Robert Gramling, Kevin Fiscella and Ronald Epstein. 2016. Eloquent silences: A musical and lexical analysis of conversation between oncologists and their patients. *Patient Education and Counselling* 99(10). 1584–1594.

Barton, Ellen. 2004. Discourse methods and critical practice in professional communication: the front-stage and back-stage discourse of prognosis in medicine. *Journal of Business and Technical Communication* 18. 67–111.

Barton, Ellen. 2006. Trajectories of alignment and the situated ethics of end-of-life discussions in American medicine. *Linguistic Insights*, 23–42. Bern: Peter Lang.

Barton, Ellen. 2007a. Institutional policies, professional practices, and the discourse of end-of-life discussions in American medicine. *Journal of Applied Linguistics* 2 (2005). 249–267.

Barton, Ellen. 2007b. Situating end-of-life decision making in a hybrid ethical frame. *Communication and Medicine* 4(2). 131–140.

Barton, Ellen. 2007c. 'Quality-of-life to the end'. *Communication and Medicine* 4(1). 121–123.

Barton, Ellen, Matthew Aldridge, Thomas Trimble and Justin Vidovic. 2005. Structure and variation in end-of-life discussions in the surgical intensive care unit. *Communication and Medicine* 2. 1–21.

Beach, Wayne A. 1990. On (not) observing behavior interactionally. *Western Journal of Speech Communication* 54. 603–612.

Beach, Wayne A. 1993. Transitional regularities for 'casual' "okay" usages. *Journal of Pragmatics* 19. 325–332.

Beach, Wayne A. 1995. Preserving and constraining options: 'Okays' and 'official' priorities in medical interviews. In G. H. Morris and Ronald J. Chenail (eds.), *Talk of the clinic: Explorations in the analysis of medical and therapeutic discourse*, 259–289. Hillsdale, NJ: Lawrence Erlbaum.

Beach, Wayne A. 2001. Diagnosing 'Lay diagnosis'. *Text* 21 (1/2). 13–18.

Beach, Wayne A. and Terri R. Metzger. 1997. Claiming insufficient knowledge. *Human Communication Research* 23(4). 562–588.

Bélanger, Emmanuelle, Charo Rodríguez, Danielle Groleau, France Légaré, Mary Ellen Macdonald and Robert Marchand. 2014. Initiating decision-making conversations in Palliative Care: an ethnographic discourse analysis. *BMI Palliative Care* 13(63). 1–12.

Bernacki, Rachelle E., Susan D. Block, American College of Physicians High Value Care Task Force. 2014. Communication about serious illness care goals: a review and synthesis of best practices. *JAMA Internal Medicine* 174(12). 1994–2003.

Benzein, Eva, Astrid Nordberg and Britt-Inger Saveman. 2001. The meaning of the lived experience of hope in patients with cancer in palliative home care. *Palliative Medicine* 15. 117–126.

Bigi, Sarah. 2011. The persuasive role of ethos in doctor-patient interactions. *Communication & Medicine* 8(1). 67–75.

Bilmes, Jack. 1985. "Why that now?" Two kinds of conversational meaning. *Discourse Processes* 8(3). 319–355.

Boden, Deidre and Donald H. Zimmerman. 1991. Structure-in-action: An introduction. In Deidre Boden and Donald H. Zimmerman (eds.), *Talk and social structure: Studies in ethnomethodology and conversation analysis*, 3–21. Berkeley: University of California Press.

Bolden, Galina. 2006. Little words that matter: Discourse markers 'so' and 'oh' and the doing of other-attentiveness in social interaction. *Journal of Communication* 56(4). 661–688.

Bolden, Galina. 2009. Implementing incipient actions: The discourse marker 'so' in English conversation. *Journal of Pragmatics* 41(5). 974–998.

Bolden, Galina. 2010. 'Articulating the unsaid' via and-prefaced formulations of others' talk. *Discourse Studies* 12(1). 5–32.

Boyd, Elizabeth A. and John Heritage. 2006. Taking the history: Questioning during comprehensive history-taking. In John Heritage and Douglas W. Maynard (eds.), *Communication in medical care. Interaction between primary care physicians and patients*, 151–184. Cambridge: Cambridge University Press.

Brown, Penelope and Stephen Levinson. 1987. *Politeness: Some universals in language usage.* Cambridge: Cambridge University Press.

van Brussel, Leen and Nico Carpentier. 2012. The discursive construction of the good death and the dying person: A discourse-theoretical analysis of Belgian newspaper articles on medical end-of-life decision making. *Journal of Languages and Politics* 11(4). 479–499.

Bucholtz, Mary. 2000. The politics of transcription. *Journal of Pragmatics* 32(10). 1439–1465.

Butow, P.N., S. Dowsett, R. Hagerty, and M. H. Tattersall. 2002. Communicating prognosis to patients with metastatic disease: What do they really want to know? *Support Care Cancer* 10. 161–168.

Button, Graham and Neil Casey. 1988. Topic initiation: Business-at-hand. *Research on Language and Social Interaction* 22. 61–91.

Cameron, Deborah. 2008. Talk from the top down. *Language and Communication* 28(2). 143–155.

Candrian, Carey. 2013. Taming death and the consequences of discourse. *Human Relations* 67. 53–69.

Carr, E. Summerson. 2006. "Secrets keep you sick": Metalinguistic labor in a drug treatment program for homeless women. *Language in Society* 35. 631–653.

Cassell, Joan. 2005. *Life and death in intensive care.* Philadelphia: Temple University Press.

Chabner, Davi-Ellen. 1996. *The Language of medicine: A write-in text explaining medical terms.* Philadelphia: W.B. Saunders.

Chafe, Wallace and Johanna Nichols. 1986. *Evidentiality: The linguistic coding of epistemology.* Norwood, NJ: Ablex.

Chatwin, John. 2008. Pre-empting 'trouble' in the homoeopathic consultation. *Journal of Pragmatics* 40(2). 244–256.

Chapman, Richard and Jonathan Gavrin. 1993. Suffering and its relationship to pain. *Journal of Palliative Care* 9(2). 5–13.

Chou, Wen-ying Sylvia. 2004. End-of-life discourse: an analysis of agency, coherence, and questions. Georgetown University PhD thesis.

Christakis, Nicholas. 1997. The ellipsis of prognosis in modern medical thought. *Social Sciences & Medicine* 44(3). 301–315.

Christakis, Nicholas. 1999. *Death foretold: prophecy and prognosis in medical care.* Chicago: University of Chicago Press.

Clayman, Steven. 1988. Displaying neutrality in television news interviews. *Social Problems* 3(4). 474–492.

Clayman, Steven. 2001. Answers and evasions. *Language in Society.* 30(3). 403–442.

Clemente, Ignasi. 2005. Clinicians' routine practices of non-disclosure: Prioritizing 'protection' over the information needs of adolescents with cancer. *Canadian Journal of Research Nursing.* 39(4). 18–34.

Clift, Rebecca. 2001. Meaning in interaction. The case of 'actually'. *Language* 77(2). 245–291.

Collins, Sarah, Nicky Britten and Johanna Ruusuvuori. 2007. *Patient participation in health care consultations: Qualitative perspectives.* New York: McGraw Hill.

Collins, Sarah, Paul Drew, Ian Watt, and Vikki Entwhistle. 2005. "Unilateral" and "bilateral" practitioner approaches in decision-making about treatment. *Social Science and Medicine* 61 (12). 2611–2627.

Collins, Sarah and Ivana Marková. 1999. Interaction between impaired and unimpaired speakers: Intersubjectivity and the interplay of culturally shared and situation specific knowledge. *British Journal of Social Psychology* 38(4). 339–368.

Costello, Brian A. and Felicia Roberts. 2001. Medical recommendations as joint social practice. *Health Communication* 13(3). 241–260.

Couper-Kuhlen, Elizabeth. 1992. Contextualizing discourse: The prosody of interactive repair. In Peter Auer and Aldo di Luzio (eds.), *The contextualization of language*, 337–364. Amsterdam: John Benjamins.

Couper-Kuhlen, Elizabeth. 2001. Interactional prosody: High onsets in reason-for-the-call turns. *Language in Society* 30(1). 29–53.

Couper-Kuhlen, Elizabeth. 2004. Analyzing language in interaction: The practice of 'never mind'. *English Language and Linguistics* 8(2). 207–237.

Couper-Kuhlen, Elizabeth. 2012a. Some truths and untruths about final intonation in conversational questions. In Jan-Peter de Ruiter (ed.), *Questions: Formal, functional and interactional perspectives*, 123–145. Cambridge: Cambridge University Press.

Couper-Kuhlen, Elizabeth. 2012b. Exploring affiliation in conversational complaint stories. In Anssi Peräkylä and Marja-Leena Sorjonen (eds.), *Emotion in interaction*. Oxford: Oxford University Press.

Craven, Alexandra and Jonathan Potter. 2010. Directives: Entitlement and contingency in action. *Discourse Studies* 12(4). 419–442.

Crippen, David. 2008. *End-of-life communication in the ICU: a global perspective*. New York: Springer.

Curl, Traci S. 2005. Practices in other-initiated repair resolution: The phonetic differentiation of 'repetitions'. *Discourse Processes* 39(1). 1–43.

Curl, Traci S., John K. Local, and Garreth Walker. 2006. Repetition and the prosody-pragmatics interface. *Journal of Pragmatics* 38(10). 1721–1751.

Curtis, J. Randall, Ruth Engelberg, Marjorie Wenrich, Elizabeth Nielson, Sarah Shannon, Patsy Treece, Mark Tonelli, Donald Patrick, Lynne Robins, Barbara McGrath and Gordon Rubenfeld. 2002. Studying communication about end-of-life care during the ICU family conference: Development of a framework. *Journal of Critical Care* 17. 147–160.

Curtis, J. Randall and Donald Patrick. 2001. How to discuss dying and death in the ICU. In J. Randall Curtis & Gordon Rubenfeld (eds.), *Managing death in the ICU*. 85–102. New York: Oxford University Press.

Curtis, J. Randall, Donald Patrick, Sarah Shannon, Patsy Treece, Ruth Engelberg, and Gordon Rubenfeld. 2001. The family conference as a focus to improve communication about end-of-life care in the intensive care unit. Opportunities for improvement. *Critical Care Medicine* 29. N26–N33.

Curtis, J. Randall and Gordon Rubenfeld (eds.). 2001. *Managing Death in the ICU*. Oxford: Oxford University Press.

Davidson, Judy. 1984. Subsequent versions of invitations, offers, requests, and proposals dealing with potential or actual rejection. In J. Maxwell Atkinson and John Heritage, (eds.), *Structures of social action: Studies in conversation analysis*, 102–128. Cambridge: Cambridge Unviersity Press.

Davies, Alan and Catherine Elder. 2006. *The Handbook of Applied Linguistics*. London: Blackwell.

Davis, Kathy. 1998. *Power under the microscope*. Dordrecht: Foris.

Defibaugh, Staci. 2014. Management of care or management of face: Indirectness in Nurse Practitioner/patient interactions. *Journal of Pragmatics* 67. 61–71.

DeLancey, Scott. 2001. The mirative and evidentiality. *Journal of Pragmatics* 33(3). 369–382.

Delvecchio Good, Mary-Jo, Byron J. Good, Cynthia Schaffer, and Stuart E. Lind. 1990. American oncology and the discourse on hope. *Cultural Medical Psychiatry* 14. 59–79.

Dersley, Ian and Anthony J. Wootton. 2000. Complaint sequences within antagonistic argument. *Research on Language and Social Interaction* 33(4). 375–406.

Dowbiggin, Ian. 2003. *A merciful end: the euthanasia movement in modern America*. Oxford: Oxford University Press.

Drew, Paul. 1991. Asymmetries of knowledge in conversational interactions. In Ivana Marková and Klaus Foppa (eds.), *Asymmetries in dialogue*, 29–48. Hemel Hempstead: Harvester/Wheatsheaf.

Drew, Paul. 1997. 'Open' class repair initiators in response to sequential sources of troubles in conversation. *Journal of Pragmatics* 28. 69–101.

Drew, Paul, John Chatwin, and Sarah Collins. 2001. Conversation analysis: A method for research into interactions between patients and health care professionals. *Health Expectations* 4(1). 58–70.

Drew, Paul and Elizabeth Holt. 1998a. Complainable matters. The use of idiomatic expressions in making compalints. *Social Problems* 35(4). 398–417.

Drew, Paul and Elizabeth Holt. 1998b. Figures of speech: Figurative expressions and the management of topic transition in conversation. *Language in Society* 27. 495–522.

Drew, Paul and Traci Walker. 2009. Going too far: Complaining, escalating, and disaffiliation. *Journal of Pragmatics* 41(12). 2400–2414.

Drummond, Kent and Robert Hopper. 1993. Some uses of yeah. *Research on Language and Social Interaction* 25(2). 203–212.

Dufault, K. and B. C. Martocchio. 1985. Symposium on compassionate care and the dying experience. Hope: Its spheres and dimensions. *Nursing Clinics of North America* 20. 379–391.

Dwamena, Francesca, Margaret Holmes-Rovner, Carolyn M. Gaulden, Sarah Jorgenson, Gelareh Sadigh, Alla Sikorskii, Simon Lewin, Robert C. Smith, John Coffey, Adesuwa Olomu and Michael Beasley. 2012. Interventions for providers to promote a patient-centered approach in clinical consultations. *Cochrane Database of Systematic Reviews* 12.

Dy, Sydney M., Kasey Kiley, Katherine Ast, Dale Lupu, Sally Norton, Susan MacMillan, Keela Herr, Joseph Rotella and David Casarett. 2015. Measuring what matters: top-ranked quality indicators for hospice and Palliative Care from the American Academy of Hospice and Palliative Medicine and Hospice and Palliative Nurses Association. *Journal of Pain & Symptom Management* 49(4). 773–781.

Eagan, Andy and Brian Weatherson (eds.). 2011. *Epistemic modality*. Oxford: Oxford University Press.

Egbert, Maria. 2004. Other-initiated repair and membership categorization: Some conversational events that trigger linguistic and regional membership categorization. *Journal of Pragmatics* 36(8). 1467–1498.

Eggly, Susan, Ellen Barton, Andrew Winckles, Louis Penner & Terrance Albrecht. 2017. A disparity of words: racial differences in oncologist-patient communication about cancer clinical trials. *Health Expectations* 18. 1316–1326.

Eliott, Jaklin A. and Ian N. Olver. 2007. Hope and hoping in the talk of dying cancer patients. *Social Science and Medicine* 64. 138–149.

Emanuel, Ezekiel J. and Linda L. Emanuel. 1992. Four models of the physician-patient relationship. *Journal of the American Medical Association* 267. 157–177.

Enfield, N. J. 2007. Meanings of the unmarked. How 'default' person reference does more than just refer. In N. J. Enfield & Tanya Stivers (eds.), *Person reference in interaction:*

Linguistic, cultural and social perspectives, 97–120. Cambridge: Cambridge Unviersity Press.

Enfield, N. J. 2011. Sources of asymmetry in human interaction: Enchrony, status knowledge and agency. In Tanya Stivers, Lorenza Mondada and Jakob Steensig (eds.), *The morality of knowledge in conversation*. Cambridge: Cambridge University Press.

Epstein, Ronald M., Peter Franks, Kevin Fiscella, Cleveland Shields, Sean Meldrum, Richard Kravitz and Paul Duberstein. 2015. Measuring patient-centered communication in patient-physician consultations: theoretical and practical issues. *Social Sciences and Medicine* 61(7). 1516–1528.

Epstein, Ronald M. and Richard L. Street. 2007. *Patient-centered communication in cancer care.* Bethesda, MD: National Institutes of Health.

Epstein, Ronald M. and Robert E. Gramling. 2013. What is shared in shared decision making? Complex decisions when the evidence is unclear. *Medical Care Research & Review* 70(1 Suppl). 94S–112S.

Epstein, Ronald M. and Anthony L. Back. 2015. A piece of my mind. responding to suffering. *Journal of the American Medical Assocation* 314(24). 2623–2624.

Fairclough, Norman. 1995: *Critical discourse analysis: The critical study of language.* London: Longman.

Ferrell, Betty R., Jennifer S. Temel, Sarah Temin, Erin R. Alesi, Tracy A. Balboni, Ethan M. Basch, Janice I. Firn, Judith A. Paice, Jeffrey M. Peppercorn, Tanyanika Phillips, Ellen L. Stovall, Camilla Zimmermann and Thomas J. Smith. 2017. Integration of palliative care into standard oncology care: American Society of Clinical Oncology clinical practice guideline update. *Journal of Clinical Oncololgy* 35(1). 96–112.

Festinger, Leon. 1962. Cognitive dissonance. *Scientific American* 207(4). 93–102.

Field, Marilyn J. and Christine K. Cassel (eds.). 1997. *Approaching death: improving care at the end of life.* Washington, DC: Institute of Medicine.

Fillmore, Charles J. 1997. *Lectures on deixis.* Stanford, CA: CSLI Publications.

Fisher, Sue. 1988. *In the patient's best interest: Women and the politics of medical decisions.* New Brunswick, NJ: Rutgers University Press.

Fisher, Sue. 1995. *Nursing wounds: Nurse practitioners, doctors, women patients, and the negotiation of meaning.* New Brunswick, NJ: Rutgers University Press.

Ford, Cecilia E. and Sandra A. Thompson. 1996. Interactional units in conversation: Syntactic, intonational and pragmatic resources for the management of turns. In Elinor Ochs, Emanuel A. Schegloff and Sandra A. Thompson (eds.), *Interaction and grammar*, 134–184. Cambridge: Cambridge University Press.

Foucault, Michel. 1980. *Power/knowledge: selected interviews and other writings 1972–1977.* Colin Gordon (trans.). New York: Pantheon.

Foucault, Michel. 1984. Des espaces autres, *Architecture, Mouvement, Continuité* 5. 46–49.

Fretheim, Thorstein, Nana Aba Appiah Amfo, and Ildikó Vaskó. 2011. Token-reflexive, anaphoric and deictic functions of 'here'. *Nordic Journal of Linguistics* 34(3). 239–294.

Frankel, Richard. 1984. From sentence to sequence: Understanding the medical encounter through microinteractional analysis. *Discourse Processes* 7(2). 135–170.

Frankel, Richard. 1990. Talking in interviews: A dispreference for patient-initiated questions in physician-patient encounters. In George Psathas (ed.), *Interaction competence: Studies in ethnomethodology and conversation analysis*, 231–262. Lanham, MD: University Press of America.

Gallois, Cindy, Lindy Wilmott, Ben White, Sarah Winch, Malcolm Parker, Nicholas Graves, Nicole Shepherd and Eliana Close. 2015. Futile treatment in hospital: doctors' intergroup language. *Journal of Language and Social Psychology* 34(6). 657–671.

Gardner, Rod. 2001. *When listeners talk: response tokens and listener stance*. Amsterdam: John Benjamins.

Geertz, Clifford. 1973. Thick description: Toward an interpretive theory of culture. In Clifford Geertz (ed.), *The interpretation of cultures: selected essays*, 3–30. New York: Basic Books.

Gill, Virginia Teas. 1998. Doing attributions in medical interaction: Patients' explanations for illness and doctors' responses. *Social Psychology Quarterly* 61. 342–360.

Gill, Virginia Teas and Douglas Maynard. 2006. Explaining illness: Patients' proposals and physicians' responses. In John Heritage and Douglas W. Maynard (eds.), *Communication in medical care: Interaction between primary care physicians and patients*, 115–150. Cambridge: Cambridge University Press.

Gill, Virginia Teas, Anne Pomerantz and Paul Denvir. 2010. Preemptive resistance: Patient's participation in diagnostic sense-making activities. *Sociology of Health and Illness* 32(1). 1–20.

Glenn, Phillip. 1989. Initiating shared laughter in multi-party conversations. *Western Journal of Speech Communication* 53(2). 127–149.

Glenn, Phillip. 1995. Laughing at and laughing with: Negotiations of participant alignments through conversational laughter. In Paul ten Have and George Psathas (eds.), *Situated order: Studies in the organization of talk and embodied activities*, 43–56. Washington, DC: University Press of America.

Goffman, Erving. 1959. *The presentation of self in everyday life*. New York: Doubleday.

Goffman, Erving. 1964. The neglected situation. *American Anthropologist* 66(6, part 2). 133–136.

Goffman, Erving. 1974. Frame analysis: an essay on the organization of experience. New York: Harper Row.

Goffman, Erving. 1979. Footing. *Semiotica* 2. 1–29.

Goodwin, Charles. 1987. Forgetfulness as an interactive resource. *Social Psychology Quarterly* 50(2). 115–130.

Goodwin, Charles. 2006. Retrospective and prospective orientation in the construction of argumentative moves. *Text and Talk* 26 (4–5). 443–461.

Goodwin, Charles and Alessandro Duranti. 1992. Rethinking context: An introduction. In Alessandro Duranti and Charles Goodwin (eds.), *Rethinking context: Language as an interactive phenomenon*, 1–42. Cambridge: Cambridge University Press.

Gramling, David and Robert Gramling. 2012. Laughing at the dark: tactical humor for autonomous decision-making in serious illness. *Journal of Palliative Medicine* 15(11). 170–172.

Gramling, Robert, Thomas Carroll, and Ronald Epstein. 2013a. What is known about prognostication in advanced illness. In Nathan Goldstein and R. Sean Morrison (eds.), *Evidence-based practice of palliative medicine*. Amsterdam: Elsevier Press.

Gramling, Robert, Sally Norton, Susan Ladwig, Paul Winters, Maureen Metzger, Timothy Quill and Stewart Alexander. 2013b. Latent classes of prognosis conversations in Palliative Care: a mixed-methods study. *Journal of Palliative Medicine* 16(6). 653–660.

Gramling, Robert, Sally Norton, Susan Ladwig, Maureen Metzger, Jane DeLuca, David Gramling, Daniel Schatz, Ronald Epstein, Timothy Quill and Stewart Alexander. 2013c. Direct observation of prognosis communication in Palliative Care: a descriptive study. *Journal of Pain and Symptom Management* 45(2). 202–212.

Gramling, Robert, Elizabeth Gajary-Coots, Susan Stanek, Nathalie Dougoud, Heather Pyke, Marie Thomas, Jenica Cimino, Mechelle Sanders, Stewart Alexander, Ronald Epstein,

Kevin Fiscella, David Gramling, Susan Ladwig, Wendy Anderson, Stephen Pantilat, and Sally A. Norton. 2015a. Design of, and enrollment in, the palliative care communication research initiative: a direct-observation cohort study. *BMC Palliative Care* 40. 1–14.

Gramling, Robert, Mechelle Sanders, Susan Ladwig, Sally Norton, Ronald Epstein, and Stewart Alexander. 2015b. Goal communication in palliative care decision-making consultations. *Journal of Pain and Symptom Management* 50(5). 701–706.

Gramling, Robert, Susan Stanek, Susan Ladwig, Elizabeth Gajary-Coots, Jenica Cimino, Wendy Anderson, Sally A. Norton and the AAHPM Research Committee Writing Group. 2016a. Feeling heard and understood: A patient-reported quality measure for the inpatient palliative care setting. *Journal of Pain and Symptom Management.* 51(2). 150–154.

Gramling, Robert, Kevin Fiscella, Guibo Xing, Michael Hoerger, Paul Duberstein, Sandy Plumb, Supriya Mohile, Joshua J. Fenton, Daniel J. Tancredi, Richard L. Kravitz, and Ronald L. Epstein. 2016b. Determinants of patient-oncologist prognostic discordance in advanced cancer. *JAMA Oncololgy* 2(11). 1421–1426.

Gramling, Robert, Susan Stanek, Paul K. Han, Paul Duberstein, Timothy E. Quill, Stewart Alexander, Wendy G. Anderson, Susan Ladwig, and Sally A. Norton. 2017. Distress due to prognostic uncertainty in palliative care: frequency, distribution and outcomes among hospitalized patients with advanced cancer. *Journal of Palliative Medicine* 21(3). 315–321.

Grice, H. Paul. 1975. Logic and conversation. In Peter Cole and Jerry L. Morgan (eds.), *Syntax and Semantics. Vol. 3, Speech Acts*, 41–58. New York: Academic Press.

Gwande, Atul. 2014. *Being mortal: medicine and what matters in the end*. New York: Metropolitan Books.

Haakana, Markku. 2001. Laughter as a patient's resource: Dealing with delicate aspects of a medical interaction. *Text* 2(1/2). 187–219.

Haakana, Markku. 2002. Laughter in medical interaction: From quantification to analysis and back. *Journal of Sociolinguistics* 6(2). 207–235.

Haakana, Markku. 2012. Laughter in conversation: The case of 'fake' laughter. In Anssi Peräkylä and Marja-Leena Sorjonen (eds.), *Emotion in interaction*, 174–194. Oxford: Oxford University Press.

Hacohen, Gonen and Emanuel A. Schegloff. 2006. On the preference for minimization in referring to persons: Evidence from Hebrew Conversation. *Journal of Pragmatics* 38(8). 1305–1312.

Hagerty, Rebecca G., Phyllis N. Butow, Peter M. Ellis, Elizabeth A. Lobb, Susan C. Pendlebury, Natasha Leighl, Craig MacLeod, and Martin H. N. Tattersall. 2005. Communicating with realism and hope: Incurable cancer patients' views on the disclosure of prognosis. *Journal of Clinical Oncology* 23. 1278–1288.

Hamel, Liz, Bryan Wu, and Mollyann Brodie. 2017. *Views and experiences with end of life medical care in Japan, Italy, the United States and Brazil: a cross-country survey*. Published by the Kaiser Family Foundation and the *Economist* magazine.

Hamilton, Heidi and Wen-Ying Sylvia Chou (eds.). 2016. *The Routledge Handbook of Language and Health Communication*. London: Routledge.

Han, Paul K., William M. Klein, and Neeraj K. Arora. 2011. Varieties of uncertainty in health care: a conceptual taxonomy. *Medical Decision Making* 31(6). 828–838.

ten Have, Paul. 1991. Talk and institution: a reconsideration of the "asymmetry" of doctor-patient interaction. In Deirdre Boden and Don H. Zimmerman (eds.), *Talk and social structure: studies in ethnomethodology and converation analysis*, 138–163. Cambridge: Polity Press.

Heath, Christian. 1992. The delivery and reception of diagnosis in the general-practice consultation. In Paul Drew and John Heritage (eds.), *Talk at work: interaction in institutional settings*, 235–267. Cambridge: Cambridge University Press.

Heath, Christian. 1989. Pain talk: The expression of suffering in the medical consultation. *Social Psychology Quarterly* 52(2). 113–125.

Heeschen, Claus and Emanuel A. Schegloff. 1999. Agrammatism, adaption theory, conversation analysis: On the role of so-called telegraphic style in talk-in-interaction. *Aphasiology* 13(4/5). 365–405.

Heft, Paul R. 2005. Necessary collusion: Prognostic communication with advanced cancer patients. *Journal of Clinical Oncology* 23(13). 3146–3150.

Heritage, John. 1998. Oh-prefaced responses to inquiry. *Language in Society* 27(3). 291–334.

Heritage, John. 2002. The limits of questioning: Negative interrogatives and hostile question content. *Journal of Pragmatics* 34(10–11). 1427–1446.

Heritage, John. 2010. Questioning in medicine. In Alice F. Freed and Susan Ehrlich (eds.), *"Why do you ask": The function of questions in institutional discourse*. 42–68. Oxford: Oxford University Press.

Heritage, John. 2012. The epistemic engine: Sequence organization and territories of knowledge. *Research on Language and Social Interaction* 45. 25–50.

Heritage, John and Douglas Maynard. 2006. Problems and prospects in the study of physician-patient interaction: 30 years of research. *Annual Review of Sociology* 32. 351–374.

Herndl, Carl and Cynthia Nahrwold. 2000. Research as social practice: A case study of research on technical and professional communication. *Written Communication* 17. 258–296.

Hesson, Ashley M., Issidoros Sarinopoulos, Richard M. Frankel, and Robert C. Smith. 2012. A linguistic study of patient-centered interviewing: Emergent interactional effects. *Patient Education and Counseling* 88. 373–380.

Hewett, David G., Bernadette M. Watson and Cindy Gallois. 2015. Communication between hospital doctors: Underaccommodation and interpretability. *Language and Communication* 41. 71–83.

Heyland, Daren, Graeme Rocker, Christopher O'Callaghan, Peter Dodek, and Deborah Cook. 2003. Dying in the ICU: Perspectives of family members. *Chest* 124. 392–397.

Horne, Rob, John Weinman, Nick Barber, Rachel Elliot, and Myfanwy Morgan. 2005. *Concordance, adherence and compliance in medicine taking. Report for the national coordianting centre for NHS service delivery and organisation R and D*. London: NCCSDO.

Hudak, Pamela, Virginia Teas Gill, Jeffrey Aguinaldo, Shannon Clark and Richard Frankel. 2010. "I've heard wonderful things about you": How patients compliment surgeons. *Sociology of Health and Illness* 32(5). 777–797.

Huddleston, Rodney. 1994. The contrast between interrogatives and questions. *Journal of Linguistics* 30(2). 411–439.

Hyde, Michael J. and Kenneth Rufo. 2001. The call of conscience, rhetorical interruptions, and the euthanasia debate. *Journal of Applied Communication Research* 28(1). 1–23.

Hymes Dell. 1972a. On communicative competence. In John B. Pride and Janet Holmes (eds.), *Sociolinguistics*. 269–285. Harmondsworth: Penguin.

Hymes, Dell. 1972b. Models of the interaction of language and social life. In John Gumperz and Dell Hymes (eds.), *Directions in sociolinguistics*, 35–71. New York: Holt, Rinehard, and Winston.

Iedema, Rick, Ros Sorensen, Jeffrey Braithwaite, and Elizabeth Turnball. 2004. Speaking about dying in the intensive care unit, and its implications for multidisciplinary end-of-life care. *Communication and Medicine* 1. 85–96.

Institutes of Medicine. 2014. *Dying in America: Improving quality and honoring individual preferences near end-of-life*. Washington, DC: The National Academies Press.

Jaén, Carlos Roberto, Robert L. Ferrer, William L. Miller, Raymond F. Palmer, Robert Wood, Marivel Davila, Elizabeth E. Stewart, Benjamin F. Crabtree, Paul A. Nutting, and Kurt C. Stange. 2010. Patient outcomes at 26 months in the patient-centered medical home national demonstration project. *Annals of Family Medicine* 8. S557–S567.

James, Deborah and Sandra Clarke. 1993. Women, men, and interruptions: A critical review. In Deborah Tannen (ed.), *Gender and conversational interaction*, 231–280. New York: Oxford University Press.

Jefferson, Gail. 1973. A case of precision timing in ordinary conversation: Overlapped tag-positioned address terms in closing sequences. *Semiotica* 9. 47–96.

Jefferson, Gail. 1974. Error correction as an interactional resource. *Language in Society* 3(2). 181–199.

Jefferson, Gail. 1983. Issues in the transcription of naturally-occurring talk: Caricature vs. capturing pronounciational particulars. *Tilburg papers in language and literature* 34.

Jefferson, Gail. 1989. Preliminary notes on a possible metric which provides for a 'standard maximum' silences of approximately one second in conversation. In Derek Roger and Peter Bull (eds.), *Conversation: An interdiscciplinary perspective*, 166–196. Clevedon, UK: Multilingual Matters.

Jefferson, Gail. 2002. Is "no" an acknowledgment token? Comparing American and British uses of (+) (-) tokens. *Journal of Pragmatics* 34. 1345–1383.

Jefferson, Gail. 2004. Glossary of transcript symbols with an introduction. In Gene H. Lerner (ed.), *Conversation analysis: studies from the first generation*, 13–31. Amsterdam: John Benjamins.

Johnstone, Barbara. 2000. *Qualitative methods in sociolinguistics*. New York: Oxford University Press.

Johnson, Marie F., Michael Lin, Saurabh Mangalik, Donald J. Murphy, and Andrew M. Kramer. 2000. Patients' perceptions of physicians' recommendations for comfort care differ by patient age and gender. *Journal of General Internal Medicine* 15. 248–255.

Jones, Charlotte M. 2001. Missing assessments: Lay and professional orientations in medical interviews. *Text* 21. 113–150.

Jones, Charlotte M. and Wayne A. Beach. 2005. Patient's attempts and doctors' responses to premature solicitation of diagnostic information. In Judith F. Duchan and Dana Kovarsky (eds.), *Diagnosis as cultural practice*, 103–136. New York: Mouton de Gruyter.

Kagawa-Singer, Marjorie and Leslie Blackhall. 2001. Negotiating cross-cultural issues at the end of life. *Journal of the American Medical Association* 286. 2993–3001.

Kamal, Arif H., Janet H. Bull, Keith M. Swetz, Steven P. Wolf, Tait D. Shanafelt, and Evan R. Myers. 2017. Future of the palliative care workforce: preview to an impending crisis. *American Journal of Medicine* 130(2). 113–114.

Kamal, Arif H., Janet H. Bull, Steven P. Wolf, Keith M. Swetz, Tait D. Shanafelt, Katherine Ast, Dio Kavalieratos, Christian T. Sinclair, and Amy P. Abernethy. 2016. Prevalence and predictors of burnout among hospice and palliative care clinicians in the US. *Journal of Pain and Symptom Management* 51(4). 690–696.

Kamio, Akio. 1997. *Territory of information*. Amsterdam: John Benjamins.

Kinmonth, Ann Louise, Alison Woodcock, Simon Griffin, Nicki Spiegal, and Michael J. Campbell. 1998. Randomised controlled trial of patient-centred care of diabetes in general practice: impact on current well-being and future disease risk. *British Medical Journal* 317. 1202–1208.

Kirchhoff, Karin, Lee Walter, Ann Hutton, Vicki Spuhler, Beth Vaughan Cole, and Terry Clemmer. 2002. The vortex: families' experiences with death in the intensive care unit. *Journal of Critical Care* 11. 200–209.

Kaufman, Sharon. 2005. *... And a time to die: how American hospitals shape the end of life*. New York: Scribner.

Kavalieratos, Dio, Jennifer Corbelli, Di Zhang, J. Nicholas Dionne-Odom, Natalie C. Ernecoff, Janel Hanmer, Zachariah P. Hoydich, Dara Z. Ikejiani, Michele Klein-Fedyshin, Camilia Zimmermann, Sally C. Morton, Robert M. Arnold, Lucas Heller, and Yael Schenker. 2016. Association between palliative care and patient and caregiver outcomes: a systematic review and meta-analysis. *JAMA* 316(20). 2104–2114.

Keeley, Maureen P. and Julie M. Jingling. 2007. *Final conversations: Helping the living and the dying talk to each other*. Acton, MA: Van de Wyk and Burnham.

Koenig. Christopher J. 2011. Patient resistance as agency in treatment decisions. *Social Science and Medicine* 72. 1105–1114.

Korsch, Barbara and Vida Francis Negrete. 1972. Doctor-patient communciation. *Scientific American* 227. 66–74.

Korsch, Barbara M., Ethel K. Gozzi and Vida Francis. 1968. Gaps in doctor-patient communication. *Pediatrics* 42. 855–871.

Kulick. Don. 2005. The importance of what gets left out. *Discourse Studies* 7 (4–5). 615–624.

Kurtz, Suzanne, Jonathan Silverman, and Juliet Draper. 2004. *Teaching and learning communication skills in medicine*. Oxford: Radcliffe Medical Press.

Kushner, Tony. 2013. *Angels in America: a gay fantasia on national themes*. Revised and complete edition. Theater Communications Group.

Lamont, Elizabeth B. and Nicholas A. Christakis. 2001. Prognostic disclosure to patients with cancer near the end of life. *Annals of Internal Medicine* 134(12). 1096–1105.

Last Acts Coalition. 2002. *Means to a better end: a report on dying in America*. Princeton, NJ: Robert Wood Johnson Foundation.

Lee, Yin-Yang and Julia Lin. 2010. Do patient autonomy preferences matter? Linking patient-centered care to patient-physician relationships and health outcomes. *Social Science and Medicine* 71(10). 1811–1818.

Lerner, Gene H. 2002. Turn-sharing: The choral co-production of talk-in-interaction. In Cecilia E. Ford, Barbara A. Fox, and Sandra A. Thompson (eds.), *The language of turn and sequence*, 222–256. Oxford: Oxford University Press.

Lerner, Gene H. 2011. On the place of hesitating in delicate formulations: A turn-constructional infrastructure for collaborative indicretion. In Makoto Hayashi, Geoffrey Raymond and Jack Sidnell (eds.), *Conversational repair and human understanding*, 95–134 Cambridge: Cambridge University Press.

Levinson, Stephen C. 1992. Activity types and language. In Paul Drew and John Heritage (eds.), *Talk at work: Interaction in institutional settings*, 66–100. Cambridge: Cambridge University Press.

Levisnon, Stephen C. 2000. *Presumptive meanings: The theory of generalized conversational implicature*. Cambridge: MIT Press.

Levinson, Stephen C. 2005. Living with Manny's dangerous idea. *Discourse Studies* 7(4–5). 431–453.

Levy, Mitchell. 2001. Making a personal relationship with death. In J. Randall Curtis and Gordon Rubenfeld (eds.), *Managing death in the ICU*, 31–36. Oxford: Oxford University Press.

Li Wei. 2016. New Chinglish and the post-multilingualism challenge: translanguaging ELF in China. *Journal of English as a Lingua Franca* 5(1). 1–25.

Lindström, Anna and Ann Weatherall. 2015. Orientations to epistemics and deontics in treatment discussions. *Journal of Pragmatics* 78. 39–53.

Lindström, Anna. 2009. Projecting non-alignment in conversation: A study of the Swedish curled ja. In Jack Sidnell (ed.), *Conversation analysis: comparative perspectives*, 135–18. Cambridge: Cambridge University Press.

Lindström, Anna and Trine Heinemann. 2009. Good enough: Low-grade assessments in caregiving situations. *Research on Language and Social Interaction* 42(4). 309–328.

Local, John K. and Gareth Walker. 2008. Stance and affect in conversation. On the interplay of sequential and phonetic resources. *Text and Talk* 28(6). 723–747.

Longo, Dan, Anthony Fauci, Dennis Kasper, Stephen Hauser, J. Larry Jameson, and Joseph Loscalzo (eds). 2014. *Harrison's principles of internal medicine*. New York: McGraw-Hill.

Lukes. Steven. 1974. *Power: a radical view*. London: MacMillan.

Lupton, Deborah. 2003. *Medicine as culture. Illness, disease, and the body in Western societies*. London: Sage.

Lutfey, Karen and Douglas Maynard. 1998. Bad news in oncology: How physicians and patients talk about death and dying without using those words. *Social Psychology Quarterly* 61(4). 321–341.

Maynard, Douglas. 1991. Interaction and asymmetry in clinicial discourse. *American Journal of Sociology* 97. 448–495.

Maynard, Douglas W. and John Heritage. 2005. Conversation analysis, doctor-patient interaction and medical communication. *Medical Education* 39. 428–435.

Mishler, Elliot. 1984. *The discourse of medicine: dialectics of medical interviews*. Norwood, NJ: Ablex.

Morgan, Marcyliena. 2010. The presentation of indirectness and power in everyday life. *Journal of Pragmatics* 42. 283–291.

Monzoni, Chiara M., Roderick Duncan, Richard Grünewald, and Markus Reuber. 2010. How do neurologists discuss functional symptoms with their patients: A conversation analytic study. *Journal of Psychosomatic Research* 71. 377–383.

Moore, Darnell. 2018. *No Ashes in the Fire: Coming of Age Black and Free in America*. New York: Hachette.

Motin Goff, Galen. 2005. Building a vaccine legacy on trust. *Fred Hutch News*, www.fredhutch.org. Feb 3.

Mouffe, Chantal. 2007. *On the political*. London: Routledge.

Mularski, Richard and Molly Osborne. 2001. The changing ethics of death in the ICU. In J. Randall Curtis and Gordon Rubenfeld (eds.), *Managing death in the ICU*, 7–17. Oxford: Oxford University Press.

National Consensus Project for Quality Palliative Care. 2013. *Clinical Practice Guidelines for Quality Palliative Care*. 3rd edn.

National Institute for Clinical Excellence (NICE). 2004. *Improving supportive & palliative care for adults with cancer*. London: NICE.

Neporent, Liz. 2015. Terri Schiavo: 10 Years After Her Death 'End of Life' Debate Rages On. *Good Morning America*, March 31.

Norton, Sally A. and Karen Amann Talerico. 2000. Facilitating end-of-life decision-making: Strategies for communicating and assessing. *Journal of Gerontological Nursing* 26. 6–13.

Nowak, Peter. 2011. Synthesis of qualitative linguistic research – a pilot review integrating and generalizing findings on doctor-patient interaction. *Patient Education and Counseling* 82. 429–441.

Nussbaum, Jon F. and Carla L. Fisher. 2009. A communication model for the competent delivery of geriatric medicine. *Journal of Language and Social Psychology* 28. 190–208.

Oakley, Ann. 1980. *Women confined*. Oxford: Martin Robertson.

Park, Joseph Sung-Yul. 2017. Transnationalism as interdiscursivity: Korean managers of multinational corporations talking about mobility. *Language in Society* 46(1): 23–38.

Parsons, Talcott. 1951. *The social system*. London: Routledge and Kegan Paul.

Pendleton, David. 1983. Doctor-patient communication: a review. In David Pendleton and John Hasler (eds.), *Doctor-patient communication*, 5–56. New York: Academic Press.

Peräkylä, Annsi. 2006. Communicating and responding to diagnosis. In John Heritage and Douglas Maynard (eds.), *Communciation in medical care: Interaction between primary care physicians and patients*, 214–247. New York: Cambridge University Press.

Pilnick, Alison and Robert Dingwall. 2011. On the remarkable persistence of asymmetry in doctor/patient interaction. A critical review. *Social Science and Medicine* 72. 1374–1382.

Pollens, R. (2012) Integrating speech-language pathology services in palliative end-of-life care. *Topics in Language Disorders* 32 (2), 137–148.

Pollner, Melvin. 1987. *Mundane Reason: Reality in Everyday and Sociological Discourse*. Cambridge: Cambridge University Press.

Raho, Joseph A. 2015. Improving communication in order to mitigate intractable conflict over medical futility. *Internet Journal of Catholic Bioethics* 2(1).

Robert Wood Johnson Foundation. 1995. *Study to understand prognosis and preferences for outcomes and risks of treatment*.

Roberts, Celia and Srikant Sarangi. 2005. Theme-oriented discourse analysis. *Medical Education* 30. 632–640.

Robinson, Jeffrey D. 2003. An interactional structure of medical activities during acute visits and its implicatiosn for patients' participation. *Health Communication* 1. 27–59.

Roe, Justin W. G. and Paula Leslie. 2010. Beginning of the end? Ending the therapeutic relationship in Palliative Care. *International Journal of Speech-Language Pathology* 12(4). 304–308.

Roter, Debra. 1977. Patient participation in the patient-provider interaction: the effects of patient question asking on the quality of interaction, satisfaction and compliance. *Health Education Monographs* 5. 281–231.

Roter, Debra and Susan Larson. 2002. The Roter interaction analysis system (RIAS): utility and flexibility for analysis of medical interaction. *Patient Education and Counseling* 42. 243–251.

Sacks, Harvey. 1992. *Lectures on conversation*. Oxford: Blackwell Press.

Sacks, Harvey, Emanuel Schegloff, and Gail Jefferson. 1974. A simplest systematics for the organization of turn-taking for conversation. *Language* 50. 696–735.

Sarangi, Srikant. 2001. Editorial: On demarcating the space between 'lay expertise' and 'expert laity'. *Text* 2(1/2). 3–11.

Sarangi, Srikant and Celia Roberts. 1999. The dynamics of interactional and institutional orders in work-related settings. In Srikant Sarangi and Celia Roberts (eds.), *Talk, work, and institutional order: discourse in medical, mediation, and management settings*, 1–60. Berlin: Mouton de Gruyter.

Sardell, Aaron N. and Steven Trierweiler. 1993. Disclosing the cancer diagnosis: Procedures that influence patient hopefulness. *Cancer* 72. 3355–3365.

Schegloff, Emanuel and Harvey Sacks. 1973. Opening up closings. *Semiotica* 7. 289–327.

Schegloff, Emanuel. 1991. Reflections on talk and social structure. In Dierdre Boden and Don Zimmerman (eds.), *Talk and social structure. Studies in ethnomethodology and conversation analysis*, 44–70. Cambridge: Polity Press.

Schegloff, Emanuel. 1997. Whose text? Whose context? *Discourse and Society* 8. 165–188.

Schenker, Yael and Robert Arnold. 2017. Toward palliative care for all patients with advanced cancer. *JAMA Oncology* 3(11). 1459–1460.

Schneiderman, Lawrence, Nancy Jecker, and Albert Jonsen. 1996. Medical futility: response to critiques. *Annals of Internal Medicine* 125. 669–674.

Schiffrin, Deborah, Deborah Tannen, and Heidi Hamilton (eds.). 2001. *Handbook of discourse analysis*. Oxford: Blackwell Press.

Silverman, Jonathan, Suzanne Kurtz and Juliet Draper. 2004. *Skills for communicating with patients*. Oxford: Radcliffe Medical Press.

Slevin, M.L., S.E. Nichols, S. M. Downer, P. Wilson, T.A. Lister, S. Arnott, J. Maher, R. L. Souhami, J. S. Tobias, A.H. Goldstone, and M. Cody. 1996. Emotional support for cancer patients: What do patients really want? *British Journal of Cancer* 74. 1275–1279.

Slomka, Jacquelyn. 1992. The negotiation of death: Clinical decision making at the end of life. *Social Science & Medicine* 35. 251–259.

Solomon, Marilyn. 2005. Realizing biolethics' goals in practice: ten ways 'is' can help "ought.' *Hastings Center Report* 3. 40–47.

Stivers, Tanya. 2007. Participating in decisions about treatment: overt parent pressure for antibiotic medication in pediatric encounters. *Social Science and Medicine* 54. 1111–1130.

Stivers, Tanya, Lorenza Mondada, and Jakob Steensig (eds.), 2011. *The morality of knowledge in conversation*. Cambridge: Cambridge University Press.

Sudnow, David. 1967. *Passing on*. Englewood Cliffs, NJ: Prentice-Hall.

SUPPORT Principal Investigators. 1995. A controlled trial to improve care for seriously-ill hospitalized patients: the study to understand prognoses and preferences for outcomes and risk of treatments (SUPPORT). *Journal of the American Medical Association* 274. 1591–1598.

Tarbi, Elise. 2017. When is enough? *Journal of Palliative Medicine* 20(9). 1038.

Temel, Jennifer S., Joseph A. Greer, Alona Muzikansky, Emily R. Gallagher, Sonal Admane, Vicki A. Jackson, Constance M. Dahlin, Craig D. Blinderman, Juliet Jacobsen, William F. Pirl, J. Andrew Billings, and Thomas J. Lynch. 2010. Early palliative care for patients with metastatic non-small-cell lung cancer. *New England Journal of Medicine* 363(8). 733–742.

Temel, Jennifer S., Joseph A. Greer, Sonal Admane, Emily R. Gallagher, Vicki A. Jackson, Thomas J. Lynch, Inga T. Lennes, Constance M. Dahlin and William F. Pirl. 2011. Longitudinal perceptions of prognosis and goals of therapy in patients with metastatic non-small-cell lung cancer: results of a randomized study of early palliative care. *Journal of Clinical Oncology* 29(17). 2319–2326.

Thompson, Teresa. 2011. Hope and the act of informed dialogue: a delicate balance at end of life. *Journal of Language and Social Pychology* 30(2). 177–192.

Todd, Alexandra Dundas. 1989. *Intimate adversaries: cultural conflict between doctors and women patients*. Philadelphia: University of Pennsylvania Press.

Waitzkin, Howard. 1991. *The politics of medical encounters*. New Haven, CT: Yale University Press.

Watson, Bernadette M., Cindy Gallois, David Hewett, and Liz Jones. 2012. Culture and health care: Intergroup communciation and its consequences. In Jane Jackson (ed.), *The Routledge handbook of language and intercultural communication, 512–524*. London: Routledge.

Weeks, Jane C., Paul J. Catalano, Angel Cronin, Matthew D. Finkelman, Jennifer W. Mack, Nancy L. Keating, and Deborah Schrag. 2012. Patients' expectations about effects of chemotherapy for advanced cancer. *New England Journal of Medicine* 367(17). 1616–1625.

West, Candace. 1984a. When the doctor is a 'lady': power, status and gender in phsyician-patient encounters. *Symbolic Interaction* 7. 87–106.

West, Candace. 1984b. *Routine complications: Troubles in talk between doctors and patients*. Bloomington, IN: Indiana University Press.

Whitehead, Anne and Angela Woods (eds.). 2016. *The Edinburgh companion to the critical medical humanities*. Edinburgh University Press.

Williamson, Elizabeth. 2012. Dutch to Santorum: Pull the Plug on Euthanasia Talk. *Wall Street Journal*. March 16.

Yalom, Irvin. D. 2009. *Staring at the sun: overcoming the terror of death*. San Francisco: Jossey-Bass.

Index